Dr Shammy Noor

*To my wonderful family who have guided and inspired me
and are the sole reason for my success and happiness.*

CONTENTS

Introduction

WHY AM I WRITING THIS?

I have lived, studied and worked in the Midlands all my life. Some might say that's a little unimaginative but I rather like the Midlands. Considering this little place was the centre of the industrial revolution, its impact on the course of humanity is surely understated and undervalued. A few years ago, having only ever worked in the big city, I decided to make a change and took on a job in a small semi-rural community. I was pleasantly surprised by how interested my patients were in building relationships with me as their GP. For the first time, the patients asked me about myself, my family and my past jobs and how I was getting on. They got to know me and I got to know them. It was in this practice that I first met my delightful elderly friend Mr James.

I enjoyed the company of Mr James who was very typical of this community. A bubbly fellow, a widower of over 20 years, who had lived a full life and had plenty of stories to tell. We had only met a few times for a review of his diabetes and high blood pressure, but he had shared many fascinating tales of his younger days as a serviceman in the British Army with the Royal Engineers and he had given me his unadulterated opinion on a range of issues! Despite his 84 years of age he embarrassed me with how much physical exercise he did each week and as a doctor I can honestly say I wish more people were just like him in his attitude to his own health and wellbeing.

So why am I writing about Mr James in this book? Well, one day, he asked me for some advice. He wanted to discuss some troubling symptoms that his family had been nagging him about for a while. We talked and I examined him and we ruled out one or two illnesses over the course of a few consultations. I eventually suggested that he might be suffering from a condition called depression and that it may have been going on for some time. I was glad he had mentioned these symptoms because I had suspected this illness previously. At this point in so many consultations, I have found that no matter whether the patient may be young or old, male or female, rich or poor, the reaction can often be very similar. Mr James laughed off the suggestion and thanked me for reassuring him that he had no significant physical problem and was off on his way.

Well, being a bit of a nag myself, I did talk to Mr James about his symptoms again and we managed to open up a dialogue about it. He was as sharp as a button and asked me lots of tough questions but in the end, he figured he had nothing to lose and decided to give treatment a go. He had some counselling and a course of medicine. I have to say, I owe a huge debt of gratitude to Mr James, because he opened my eyes to the elephant in the room when he came back to tell me how he was getting on.

"I feel like I've got the real me back – for the first time in 40 years," he said. The poor fellow had lived with the burden of depression for so long, it had become part of his life. Underneath all of those symptoms of irritability and inability to enjoy the things he once enjoyed was the good old Mr James who was finally back once the burden of illness had finally been lifted. The short circuit was removed and the buzzing that had been in his brain was finally removed. Peace... at last.

Well this got me thinking. This is an intelligent, strong, delightful and interesting individual who has gotten through the thick and thin of life. He looks after himself and has pride in his own life and that of his family and community. So why was he so averse to treating the depression? When a few simple measures may have given him his life back years ago, what was it that changed his mind now?

There's a bit of me that is disappointed and a bit of me that is a little ashamed that the therapies to treat Mr James and so many millions of people like him have been around for decades. The thing that stops people from getting better from these illnesses is not the lack of drug research nor the lack of funding, but one simple and very dangerous thing: misinformation.

As a doctor, I am in the business of making people better. If I were a mechanic, people would bring their cars to me and I would use whatever skills I had learned to work out what was wrong and do my best to put it right. The first thing I might do is listen to the car owner's story. What seems to be the fault with the car? Does it come and go or is it there all the time? How long has it been faulty?

All of these questions would give me a fair idea of what the problem might be and the next thing I suppose I would do is start to examine the car. I might even run a few tests to form a diagnosis. At the end of that process I could form an opinion. After the obligatory chat with the owner about quotes and timetables I might set to work and do my best to get the car in as good condition as it can be.

In many ways, my job as a doctor isn't all that different to the mechanic. I take the history, perform an examination, I might need some confirmatory tests after which I might, if I can, form a diagnosis. Of course, my 'cars' as a doctor are human beings. Even though I regularly get asked by my patients for an M.O.T., there are, of course, one or two differences between cars and humans!

It doesn't really take much imagination to realise that the analogy between cars and people starts to break down pretty quickly (excuse the pun!). For a start, we all know what a car is supposed to look like. It comes, identical to the next, off a production line, with a set blueprint and a detailed manual. We know all about its parts; how they were made, where they were made, and how to get a new one if the old one fails. There is a definition of 'working properly' for a car – and that should be exactly how it is when it rolls out of the show room for the first time – brand new and gleaming.

But there is another slightly less obvious difference between fixing cars and fixing humans. And that is something that has become more and more apparent to me as a doctor, the more I practice. That difference is what I call the 'no-go' zone.

THE 'NO-GO' ZONE

I'm sure there are people that have fallen very much in love with their cars! I have no doubt that there are many examples of folk that love their cars like they love their families. I can certainly remember many times when I've been bored almost to a coma listening to people passionately talk about their beloved cars. But I really don't ever remember hearing of anyone that would take their cherished vehicle to the mechanic and specifically not want them to investigate a problem with a particular part of the car.

"My car is not working but please investigate

everything but the gearbox... I don't want to hear that there could be anything wrong with the gearbox. As long as the rest of the car is fine I'll take it back as it is" – sounds silly, doesn't it? Nobody puts the gearbox in the 'no-go' zone.

"I'm having all sorts of trouble with my car – funny noises, stopping in the road. Please check it out and fix it – if it's anything to do with the suspension – just hand it back and I'll get on with it as it is". I suppose this owner could be a suspension expert. But I would be pretty surprised if there were many rational explanations for going to the mechanic and saying this.

As a 'human mechanic' I hear this a lot. Many people will of course come to visit the doctor with some ideas about what their condition could be and, in my opinion, the patient's ideas are very often on the right track. Patients may also have concerns about possible diagnosis that they might have which may be more serious and- thankfully, most of the time they can be reassured that they can be ruled out. Patients have expectations that they go into a consultation with and hopefully, with the doctor, together they can meet these expectations.

But, even though we are living in the 21st century, there are still the human 'no-go' zones. That zone that I am talking about is, of course... mental illness. Depression and anxiety are definitely 'no-go'.

I think that there have been some significant improvements in attitudes towards mental health in recent years but I still think there is a lot of ground to be made up. Through this book, I will try to fathom why we, as a society, still hold onto these myths. Undoubtedly the media and Hollywood have played their part and so has the sewing circle! But I really do feel that the time is now right for us as a species and as a society of interconnected beings to finally get educated and informed about mental illness. What really is it? What isn't it? Why does it happen? How do we get rid of it and get on with our lives?

As a doctor, I see many people affected by these illnesses. Even in the 21st century, in an age of apparent enlightenment, I hear so many people tell me the same myths, old wives tales and misconceptions that were prevalent centuries ago. People can be cynical, embarrassed and even offended by the very notion that they could be suffering from depression or anxiety. Sometimes entering into a discussion about depression or anxiety as a diagnosis can result in people turning away. Many people still believe that an illness of the mind is not physical. Depression and anxiety are real and as we shall see further in the book – they are as physical as a fracture to the forearm or an infection of the kidney.

If you are reading this book you might have recently had a diagnosis of depression or anxiety, or you may feel that such an illness is contributing to other physical illnesses such as irritable bowel disease or the breathlessness felt through emphysema. You may be worried that you are suffering, currently undiagnosed, as many people unfortunately are. You may just be interested in getting to the bottom of what depression actually is and what people mean when they talk about depression, anxiety, stress or emotion. It may be that you have a loved one who has recently been diagnosed with depression or you may be concerned that a loved one is suffering but can't get to grips with it. I would be delighted if, as a result of reading this, your attitude towards mental health changes and, consequently, you will help those around you to be more enlightened too.

I hope that by writing this book I can make just a little difference in starting to change the public attitude to mental illness by exposing the myths and showing that they don't hold up to even the most basic scrutiny.

In essence, I feel that there is a major hurdle in the successful treatment of depression in our society. This is not due to a lack of treatment, nor is it a lack of medical staff to help with the disease. It certainly isn't a lack of funding for research. Resources are always scarce and as the human population of the planet grows and gets older these resources will be spread even thinner. But the treatments and resources are already here, so why aren't some people getting better? The limiting step or the hurdle that we need to get over is ignorance. There seems little point in top scientists and doctors developing new breakthrough drugs and therapies if they are shunned by the very people that could benefit the most from them.

THE IMMUNISATION EXPERIENCE

1980 was a remarkable year in medical history. In this year, the disease smallpox was declared as eradicated from the globe. Humans had beaten this deadly disease that, for centuries, had claimed the lives of millions.

In-fact a type of smallpox 'vaccine' was first described and widely used by Chinese doctors in the 10th century AD. The people of the time had realised that anyone who had previously been infected with smallpox and survived the disease never went on to have the illness again. Chinese physicians found that by taking powdered scabs from individuals with smallpox and applying it to the skin of others, they could induce a mild case of the illness and the individual would never suffer smallpox for the rest of their life. During the 17th and 18th century, this technique, now called 'variolation', was in widespread use in China, India and Turkey. From Turkey, it spread to Europe and the Americas. The type of vaccination that we recognise today was first pioneered by a British physician named Edward Jenner. He discovered that you didn't need to use smallpox but even exposure to the much milder cowpox would confer immunity. Better, safer and more effective vaccines followed until the last known naturally occurring diagnosis of smallpox was recorded in Somalia in 1977.

In the early days of immunisation, there was widespread fear, misconception and opposition. This came from politicians, religious leaders and many in the medical profession. The objections were on grounds of medical safety, mistrust of the effectiveness and moral opposition. The moral issue being that God had sent disease to punish those that had sinned and as such, man should not seek to eradicate Gods means of punishment. So, despite there being the existence of treatments to prevent this disease, smallpox continued to be rife amongst communities.

So, what has all this got to do with the treatment of mental health illness? Well, on the face of it, it doesn't seem like much at all. However, there is one very strong and important link. The single biggest factor in the success of immunisation programs has been the acceptance of it in society as a whole. Before the understanding of the treatment and prevention process whole populations would fail to receive the vaccines, despite the fact that the vaccines were available. Even in the modern era, health scares appear – most notably the recent association of the MMR vaccine and cases of autism. This resulted in many people being misinformed about the true values and dangers of immunisation. Once again, diseases that were perfectly treatable and preventable started to rise up again. Measles cases steadily rose in the early parts of this century. The reason was not that the vaccines were not available or not properly administered, but simply that the public's perception of the illness and treatments changed. Misinformation was the cause of worsening illness.

Mr James did not get the treatment for his depression, not because the treatment wasn't there but because of the misunderstanding and misconception that existed in the society around him which actively prevented him from seeking and receiving help. Just as with immunisation, there is little benefit in just having the treatments exist. The true value of these can only be realised when society understands and accepts the benefits.

This book won't be a medical textbook although I have

tried to include lots of scientific details of this illness where it is informative and interesting. Nor is this book a manual of diagnosis or treatment. I have no doubt that many experts in the field will sit on either side of some of the debates raised. Nothing in this book will replace going to speak to your own doctor about any health concerns that you have.

However, I hope this book can achieve some success in trying to explain the disease concepts through analogy that all intelligent laypeople can relate to and understand. Everyone knows what a fracture is. If someone says that they have broken a bone, there aren't many things that they can mean. An orthopaedic surgeon might disagree, by telling me that there are many types of broken bone. But a group of average laypeople would all pretty much agree with what a broken bone is. In this day and age, I think we all know what an infection is. Viruses and bacteria are all part of our basic education and if someone was to say they had a urinary infection, I think it's fair to say that an average group people would all agree on the meaning of this.

Ask for an explanation of depression though, or anxiety or stress, and you'd be hard pushed to find two sets of answers the same. We all have our prejudices about these illnesses and we all have misconceptions – but hopefully, if I achieve what I set out to, we can all start to treat these simple but potentially devastating illnesses with the same degree of education as we do with all the others. And, at the end of it all, we can all live healthier and happier lives.

THE JOURNEY OF THIS BOOK

If this book is to achieve its aim it must do a number of things. I hope to be able to address these one by one and I endeavour to leave you, the reader, with a fresh new insight into this mysterious and misunderstood disease.

This book will ask and answer the questions outlined below. It would be a useful exercise to mentally ask yourself these questions before reading the book. At the end, ask them again. Will anything have changed or become clearer?

Part 1

"What is depression?"

This must be dealt with first. Here, we will define the illness. This won't be a detailed pathological insight but it will give a clear overview of what we are dealing with. This will help focus where our energies are needed. This is the 'Short Circuit'.

Part 2

"Why do I feel the way I feel?"

In this section, we will explore the difference between stress, personality and illness. It will hopefully become clear that depression is distinct from but related to life pressure and how strength of character and personality has nothing to do with it.

Part 3

"Why does society think the way it does about this illness?"

It is not enough to simply say that society is ignorant about mental health illness. There are good reasons for why people think and feel the way they do about this illness and in this chapter, we will explore these reasons.

Part 4

"What can we do about it?"

Finally, now that we have a better concept of what this illness is, we can start to beat it. In this chapter I will discuss a range of possible methods to help.

Let's get started.

Part 1 - What is depression?

WHAT IS DEPRESSION?

"Seeing isn't believing. Believing is seeing."

Little Elf Judy, The Santa Claus (1994)

If we see something, we believe it. However, if we don't believe it, we may never see it. This is the perpetual problem with societal attitude toward mental health illness. If this book is to make a difference, it must break this cycle.

Imagine being the first person to tell ancient surgeons that cleanliness was the key to reducing infection rates in their patients. It would have probably sounded ridiculous. Almost like saying that washing your hands would somehow cure you of cancer. But what if you were able to show them, through some ancient microscope, the colonies of bacteria that line the surface of their patients' wounds. And then show them how, after washing, there seems to be far fewer bacteria and the patient fared much better. Now you would have an audience listening to you. Let's apply this theoretical microscope to the subject of depression to see exactly what it is – and we may find that it is really not that mysterious at all.

A significant part of society's misunderstandings of depression lies in the fact that the condition is poorly explained by medical science. And when the medical scientists can't agree it is likely that doctors, whose job is to translate medical science into practical improvements in health, will have widely different ways of looking at this illness. However, there are, I feel, ways to frame the condition in such a way that it makes sense to most people. This is where this book comes in and will try to be different.

What has come before this hasn't worked in helping people understand. The public are as misinformed now as they were decades ago. Society has moved on in so many ways in the last half century but the subject of depression and mental health as a whole remains somewhat backwards in comparison. It does not need much of a trip back in time to find attitudes and behaviours that we would consider appalling in today's age. The subjects of race, sexuality and gender are no longer subject to the widespread institutionalised bigotry and prejudice that they were a generation ago, although sadly it does still exist. Why has the treatment of mental illness not followed the same pattern? We need a new way in which to model, describe and explain the illness.

This book attempts to do just that. If my patients' reactions and responses are anything to go by I can safely say that this new explanation will be well received, understandable and will robustly explain so many seemingly paradoxical issues with depression. If this new explanation is to make sense, it must be consistent with a number of observations about depression and those who suffer it.

Firstly, it must show how despite being a strong and powerful character, depression can still strike, such as in the case of Winston Churchill. Then, it must explain how and why depression can exist even in those people who have money, fame and every conceivable worldly privilege. Finally, it must explain the myriad of symptoms that are seen in people with this terrible affliction. Whilst a sense of sadness is present in those who suffer depression, there is also fear, difficulty in concentration, an inability to find joy in otherwise enjoyable activities, anger, sleep disturbance, appetite changes, relationship difficulties, memory loss, fatigue and a loss of self-worth amongst a myriad of other symptoms.

Let us see if the short circuit explanation can deliver on this task.

THE SHORT CIRCUIT

Our brains are complex, very complex. In terms of interconnections, the human brain is the most complex entity in the known universe. Furthermore, neuroscientists are only just starting to grasp the basics of how this enormously complex mass of biological material can perform intelligent tasks almost instantaneously that no supercomputer in the world can match. OK, so we can devise a machine to play chess to beat a grandmaster. And we can build a machine to model the conditions at the beginning of time and create hypotheses about it. But ask each of those machines to drive a car, or make some toast or colour in a children's puzzle book or even swap jobs with each other and they fail hopelessly. It will be quite some time before anyone can claim to have understood the human brain.

Whilst the molecular biology and chemistry of thoughts may still be a complete mystery, we can talk with a little more confidence about how we process these thoughts. It is a fault in this processing that explains many mental illnesses.

Let's get straight in and consider what exactly depression or anxiety really is.

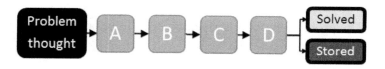

Look at the diagram above. This is how we normally process a thought. It starts at point A, moves to B then to C and D etc. There is a linear workflow. If we consider problems that appear in our lives, these may start a thought process – let's call this a 'problem thought'. The problem could be little or large. It could be "My house is being repossessed", or it could be "What have I done with my car keys". The nature of the problem can be vastly varied and therefore the 'problem thought' can be vastly varied. The problem could be about something in the past, the present or potential problems in the near or distant future. We all have these problem thoughts, some more than others and more at certain times in our lives than others.

However, when there is a normal work flow process, the problem thought progresses along the production line. The problem may be solved by the end, in which case the thought disappears and is stored in memory. Many problems are much more difficult to solve, and these problem thoughts may spend longer in the workflow. Often, when the problem thought comes to its conclusion, if it is not solved, it may be put in 'storage'. The problem thought will come back in at point A when it next needs to be considered. This could be the following day, later that week or in the next year – depending, of course, on the nature of the problem at hand.

Different people may 'handle' these problem thoughts in different ways. Different people have different levels of resources available to them. We all have experienced different life events and as such some can manage these problem thoughts with greater efficiency than others. We all have different personalities, and we all have individual outcomes to our thought processes. No two people will have exactly the same work flow, indeed, even in the same individual, the workflow might take a different path at different times in their life. This is all normal.

The problem thoughts themselves are NOT depression. There may be many more problem thoughts at certain points in our lives but no matter how many or what the nature of these thoughts are, it is not helpful to think of the thoughts themselves as depression.

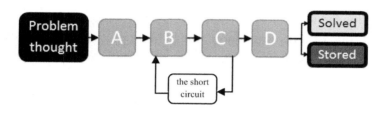

Now let's consider this altered diagram. This time the problem thought starts at point A and progresses to B and then C. However, now there has been a change in the workflow. From C, the problem thought gets 'short-circuited' back to B. It then passes back to C, followed by B, then C, B, C, B. It's now stuck. The problem thought simply bounces. It has no destination, and there is no rationality to it being in the workflow. The thought lingers, it ruminates, persistently batting back and forth from B to C to B to C. The affected individual will often have minimal control over this cycle. It matters not what the problem thought is – there is the potential for it to get trapped. Equally, the existence of the short circuit is not in any way related to the affected individual's personality, intelligence or strength of character. This is a fault that can appear in anyone at any time. Just like any other illness.

This is depression. Depression, therefore, is not the fact that problem thoughts exist – we all have these – some more than others. But, in fact, it is simply the short circuit that causes the thought to be locked down into this cycle. This simple, tiny fault is to blame for a vast array of outward symptoms. Once you see the true nature of the fault these symptoms all start to make sense.

Now that we have this short-circuit in the workflow, problems start to appear. Notice also that the process can start to break down no matter what the nature of the problem thought is. People who suffer with depression will often mentally fight themselves about the fact that they have 'nothing to be depressed about'. In fact, it is a commonly held belief that only those with significant hardship are 'allowed' to suffer with the illness of depression. Looking at the illness as a short-circuit now makes more sense. It is quite possible to live a life full of hardship, faced with many daily unsolvable problems but because the workflow is not short circuited, the symptoms of depression don't appear. Equally, in those people living privileged and comfortable lives, if the illness strikes they will become ill. The illness shows no preference for people who live in hardship. Nor does it show much preference for anyone in particular. It can strike anywhere to anyone. You don't need anything to be 'depressed about'. The statement is as nonsensical as saying someone has 'nothing to have diabetes about' or 'nothing to have asthma about'.

The nature or severity of the problem, and therefore the problem thought in some respects, is irrelevant. Once the short-circuit fault exists, anything can get stuck. The problem thoughts that tend to get stuck can vary from person to person however. These can range from incidents many years in the past, sometimes they are the most trivial or irrelevant details whilst other times they are very major issues in the individual's life at the time. When we think of helping fix depression, we mustn't get too side-tracked with the problem thought itself. The issue may sometimes be completely unfixable or so far in the past that nothing can be done about it anyway. It is very common to believe that the only way an individual can be cured is for the problem thought itself to be solved. However, what can be fixed is the short circuit. If we can get the workflow going again, no matter what the problem, it will progress through to some logical end point. That end point may not be the complete solution to the problem but at least it won't be stuck. The ruminations will stop. Thinking will be more logical, more constructive and less all consuming.

So now we are looking at depression in a new way. It no

longer represents the magnitude of problems in a person's life – that may or may not be there. Nor does it represent an individual's personality – anyone has the right to analyse thoughts in their own way. However, depression, in a nutshell, is the short circuit that exists in the thought processing machinery. This is an illness, like any other illness. Just like asthma is a tightening of the airways or diabetes is a fault with the processing of glucose, so depression is a rational, demonstrable fault of an organ of the body – the mind.

Think of listening to a terrible news story on the radio. This can be a story that induces sadness, anger, fear or frustration. Now imagine the news story repeats itself over and over every 30 seconds. The radio itself is now stuck on repeat. The news story is now heard over and over. The emotion this induces is now magnified and can become overwhelming. It can be tempting to believe that the only way out is for the problem of the news story to be addressed in some way. This will of course help. But we must also fix the radio. If this is not done, then the next news story will become stuck and have the same effect over and over again. Fixing the radio does not, of course, change the news or the world. But it will allow the workflow to restart. The problem is still there but it does not cause the crippling symptoms it once did.

THE SYMPTOMS OF THE SHORT CIRCUIT

I have often thought that maybe 'depression' needs to change its name. The word often conjures so much prejudice and is associated with so much misinformation that it has become an almost useless term to use without thorough explanation. Not only that, but I'm not sure that even once we get through the misinformation, that the word is a particularly good representation of what I have described above. Maybe 'thought process disorder' would be a better name or maybe 'workflow error illness'. I'd better leave thinking of a name to those with a more creative imagination!

But let's consider what the effects of this error are.

Consider the individual, whose thoughts are on lockdown. Problem thoughts never get past point C. Forever bouncing from B to C to B to C. Many people who suffer with depression or anxiety can relate to this. Hours go by and the same thought may be floating around and around. We will call this a rumination. Then another problem thought may appear at point A. This too may never reach point D, forever trapped between B and C. People will sometimes realise this is happening. An inner voice from the back of the head will appear saying 'stop it, stop going over this again and again'. This inner voice may succeed for a period of time but after a while the ruminations will start up again.

Now the individual's brain is giving a disproportionately large amount of energy to this process. This then becomes like a bee, buzzing in the head, unremitting. Now it's more difficult to concentrate. When trying to engage in communication with other people, there is a constant distraction. Irritability and anger ensues and it becomes difficult to remember details of conversations. Things which would normally be enjoyable are no longer so. How can you enjoy your favourite TV show, your round of golf or your time with the grandchildren with the constant unrelenting buzzing in the brain? Furthermore, sleep is disturbed and fitful and many people find themselves wake early in the morning when the buzzing begins again. These are all the effects of the short circuit on the brain's ability to do all its other jobs. And as a result, all of these other jobs suffer.

But this is not all. The nature of the rumination itself is important. You may have noticed that at points in this book I have used the term depression or anxiety interchangeably. In fact, these two syndromes share the exact same cause when you look at the short circuit explanation. The only difference is that in those suffering with depression, the problem thoughts that are locked in are about bad things that have already happened. In those suffering with anxiety, the problem thoughts are about bad things that may happen in the future. The underlying problem, the error of processing, is the exact same short circuit that prevents thoughts from progressing through the workflow in a productive and rational fashion.

DEPRESSION OR ANXIETY?

Many people will have a bit of both. When looked at from this point of view, it is fairly easy to see how the two things are not only related but in fact on a pathological level, they are really just variations of the exact same thing. This does a lot to explain why treatments for one are equally effective for the other. Let's consider how the nature of the problem thought will produce more specific symptoms.

Take an individual whose ruminating problem thoughts are about bad things that have already happened. It may be relationships haunting them from the past or even the most insignificant trivial issues in their lives now. This person will have a feeling of loss and sadness. They may feel angry or personally hurt. The range of emotion associated with depression is vast. Loneliness, insecurity, hopelessness, futility of future actions and damaged self-worth. The despair associated with this illness must not be misunderstood or underestimated. It is the greatest peril of society not to recognise this suffering as this in itself magnifies the situation. Later in this book we will see that this is actually one of the most lethal diseases, accounting for the deaths of more young people than any other medical complaint. Added to this, the person suffering has no concept of why this is happening. Why are they experiencing this overwhelming emotion? 'Am I going mad?' they might ask themselves. When people experience depression and they are ruminating about a problem thought that has no obvious solution, such as a bereavement, it can feel that situation has no resolution. How can they ever feel better unless their loved one comes back? How can they get out of this evil storm whilst they are still being bullied at work? Not only is this mentally exhausting, it is physically draining too. Depression is one of the biggest causes of persistent unexplainable fatigue. It can result in a weakened immune system with the sufferer picking up niggling minor infections recurrently. It is indeed a bleak place.

Thankfully, the cause of the despair is not wholly down to the problems. It is in fact the short circuit that is doing it. And this can be fixed. Once fixed the problem thoughts will still appear, however they will flow and not get trapped. There will be relief.

On the other hand, what if the problem thoughts are about something bad that is about to happen? "What if my son doesn't come home?", "The aeroplane might come down in the sky," or "This mark must be cancer". This person will be nervous. They will have fear and panic. They will be obsessive about trying to stop the bad events from playing out. They may be extra vigilant and wary. Like the depressed person, they may feel angry, insecure and out of control. The outward appearance of those suffering predominantly with depression compared to those with anxiety may be remarkably different. And this is probably the reason that the two illnesses are not often considered together but, as has been explained, they share the very same underlying core issue. However, with just a little change in the character of the problem thought, the effect further downstream can be huge. Like depression, anxiety can also be associated with a number of symptoms affecting various organs of the body. One of the primary defence mechanisms of the body is to prepare for *flight or fight* when it senses danger. This involves the release of adrenaline. The heart beats faster; palpitations are felt; breathlessness can be experienced. Many people describe pins and needles sensations in their fingers and toes. On top of this, the physical symptoms themselves can start a new ruminating problem thought – further exacerbating the problem.

Many people who suffer this sort of illness will describe symptoms of depression and anxiety. In some it can be a roughly even split of the two whilst in others it is predominantly one or the other. Whilst the outward appearance may be different, there really isn't much distinction to be made. They are really just different flavours of the same thing.

The principle aim in treating patients is to close the short circuit. No treatment can solve every problem in people's lives. Medical treatment does nothing to solve poverty, bereavement, housing or employment issues. But let's remember that depression and anxiety are not the existence of these things. They are illnesses of the processing of the mind. They can be treated. Once they are controlled, people get their personality back. They get their ability to concentrate, their ability to relate to others, their ability to enjoy and their ability to think back. The buzzing in the brain abates. It is a fundamental right of any person who has been disabled by illness, whether physically or psychologically, to be treated with respect and compassion. Especially when the illness is treatable.

THE PROBLEM OF INSIGHT

There is another peculiarity about mental illness over other forms of illness: the loss of insight. Imagine an illness that made you believe that you did not have it. There are many examples in the biology of viruses or bacteria that, once they infect another organism, go about making changes to the host that dampens its ability to detect the invader. In evolutionary terms, this is great for the attacker.

Towards the later stages of the twentieth century, a new deadly illness began to spread and cause terror amongst communities and eventually whole nations and continents. Although now the disease is much better understood and treatments are available which can give patients a near normal life expectancy, it remains incurable and is still responsible for millions of deaths across the globe every year. The offender is the Human Immunodeficiency Virus, HIV. This little devil owes its success to the fact that it attacks and destroys the very system in the body that would detect it and remove it. In essence, the body's own immune system eventually fails to recognise the virus which does a very clever job of hiding itself. On a cellular level, the virus has dampened the insight of the body's defences which no longer see it as foreign, abnormal or dangerous – they can't even tell whether it is there or not. This tactic of switching off the host's ability to recognise the virus as different is very effective and there are many subtly different ways in which this can happen.

Larger organisms will do this too. Consider the mosquito. At best, it's an annoying biting flying midge, at worst it is the vector for one of the biggest causes of death in human history - malaria. When it lands on the skin of its prey it injects saliva through its proboscis which contains immune material that can give it a sort of invisibility to its host. Being swatted half way through a blood meal is not particularly convenient to the mosquito and blood sucking is probably its most vulnerable time – so what better tactics than to make yourself invisible to the host.

Depression, anxiety and other forms of illness of the

mind can often reduce a person's insight. OK, they are not viruses, nor insects – but they do trick the victims mind into invisibility. There aren't many illnesses like this. When you have pneumonia, you know you are ill. There's no mistaking the pain of a heart attack or meningitis or an epileptic seizure. But when the disease is of the mind, very strange things can happen. It becomes harder and harder to know the difference between a thought process that has been created or moulded by illness and another one that is normal and real. This can be very stark in the more vivid disorders like schizophrenia. A phenomenon known as a 'delusion of reference' can lead the victim to believe that a news story on television or in a newspaper is about them specifically. The loss of insight is such that to that person the newspaper story is most definitely about them. There is no way to distinguish the scenario that the person has genuinely been written about in a news story, or the illness making them believe it. A few years ago, I watched the superb film, 'A Beautiful Mind'. In the opening sequences, we see the protagonist, the Nobel laureate John Nash involved in a tense stand-off between US department of defence special agents and Russian spies. It's gripping and the audience is wholly engrossed. It's only later in the film we realise that the entire set of events is delusional – but up until that point we would have no way of knowing that it was anything other than the absolute truth.

These are somewhat extreme examples. In the more common illnesses of depression or anxiety, the same invisibility can occur, even if it is not so dramatic. You could say that the brain is lying. I prefer not to think of it like that. The illness lies. And the illness protects itself by making itself invisible and making the brain believe that the abnormal thoughts are real. Where other people around them may see that their thoughts are changed or more irrational, they themselves may not see it. This is not because they are not intelligent enough nor because they haven't thought it through, but because the illness has in some way protected itself by reducing the person's insight. In depression, the feeling of hopelessness or worthlessness can be overwhelming. In-fact it is a lie. The devil that is the disease is talking and when the patient is better – only when the patient is better – will it become obvious that this was a lie all along.

For a person suffering with anxiety, the expected negative outcomes of a benign event can be vastly overestimated. Having another individual simply saying, "Don't be silly. Aren't you over-exaggerating the danger?" would be as nonsensical to the sufferer as saying the very same to a person stuck in a cage with a hungry tiger.

THE TINTED GLASSES

Imagine you were wearing a pair of glasses that had a red tint. But imagine also that you had no way of knowing that you were wearing these glasses. Everything around you would appear red tinged. A blue ball would appear purple. You would probably, quite rightly, disagree with another person who said that the ball was in fact blue.

Now, instead of red-tinted glasses, imagine glasses that made animals look more dangerous. Most people would agree that it is fairly rational to be afraid of poisonous snakes. If you saw a cobra, you would more than likely have a response of self-protection and fear – the *flight or fight* response. If you were completely unaware that you were wearing these special glasses, then you might find yourself responding to a harmless worm in the same way. Because the glasses were tricking your mind into believing something else, you would be behaving perfectly rationally to a perceived threat.

In many ways, mental illness can be seen as these sorts of glasses. The person behind them is not changed, they are behaving and thinking rationally but the illness has altered their perception of the world around them such that the information they receive has been altered.

WHY IS DEPRESSION SO
SUCCESSFUL?

*"the finest trick of the devil is to persuade you that he does not
exist"*

- Charles Baudelaire (1821-67)

Fans of the film 'The Usual Suspects' will recognise
this line. Chillingly delivered by Kevin Spacey playing
the twisted Verbal Kint. But what does it mean?

Theologians of the monotheistic trilogy of Judaism,
Christianity and Islam will argue that this describes the
underhand methods of the dark side of the eternal battle

between good and evil. The devil, in his mischief will deceive, imitate and cheat. Without constant awareness and wariness, his victims could easily be duped and misled by the elusive creature. Only when they recognise and capture the acts of the devil will his plans be ruined. And they will only recognise and capture his acts when they are vigilant and they look for those acts. They will only be vigilant for them when they believe the devil to be there. His best chance of pursuing his plan and evade detection would be to convince everyone that there is nothing to look for at all.

I am not a theologian. My précis above may even be insulting in its simplicity to those who profess an education in theology – I have no desire to open a debate with them. But to me as a physician and author of a book about depression, it resonates the very essence of why depression is so hard to find. You don't look for fairies at the bottom of the garden if you don't believe in fairies, you don't hunt for ghosts in the attic if you don't believe in ghosts, you don't wait up for Santa Claus once you realise he isn't real, and you don't search for illness of the mind if you don't believe in such things. Three of the examples in the previous sentence are indeed made up and one isn't. Without a doubt, the greatest trick depression ever pulled was to convince the world that it doesn't exist.

This is the concept of insight. We are dealing with an

illness so mischievous that it blinds the sufferer into believing that it's not really there. It makes the victim believe that's its symptoms are real - the barrage of negative messages, the inability to concentrate, relax or enjoy and the miserable outlook. It will make them believe that the sufferer is the source of these things, not the disease. How can it be the disease when the disease doesn't exist? This ability to destroy insight is indeed the greatest power the disease has. A cloak of invisibility. Add to this its ability to mimic and blend and we start to understand why it is so difficult to catch. Its symptoms can start out vague and mimic a number of generic non-specific viral illnesses, such as tiredness and 'flu-like' symptoms. And its mental symptoms are more likely to magnify or exaggerate a life stressor than come out and out with a blatant delusion. Schizophrenic delusions will often have an element of bizarreness about them which help them stand out as clearly abnormal. When a neighbour tells you that the voices on the TV are telling him to hide in his attic or that aliens have landed and are inserting chips into everyone's head, this is very clearly delusional. The neighbour will have no insight of course, but those around him will spot that he is ill. In depression or anxiety, the nature of the thought changes will be far more subtle. Delusion is not the right word for them because the sufferer will not be so fixed in their belief. However, the illness will be influencing the thoughts. Thoughts of worthlessness, of despair, of lack of hope and total loss of control are being seeded by the illness. Each victim will have their own personalised version of thoughts, each with total relevance to their own lives and experience. The illness will be constantly presenting 'evidence' to the victim –

'you see, you are worthless – look what happened',
'you see, they do hate you – think about what they did last year'
'you see, the world is just as bad as you thought – look what you have just seen in the newspaper"

The sufferer has no way of distinguishing these from reality. These aren't 'voices' in the head – that would be far too obvious – moreover, they are ruminations that keep recurring and going round and round. And as the depression is so thoroughly cloaked – no one will even believe that it is there. The thoughts will feel real, and they will make the sufferer increasingly ill. The person will feel that the reality that has now formed in their minds is the true picture of what is around them – and that it is them (and the world) that is bad and at fault. And it is them that is going mad. This can be crippling. The real devil, the illness, gets away undetected. It sometimes even gets away with murder.

Unfortunately, it doesn't stop there. Whilst the patient's insight is blunted, so it seems, is the insight of society as a whole. It is an unfortunate combination that an illness almost invisible to the sufferer also blinds the community in which the sufferer lives. How can people believe in the invisible, untouchable, 'non-physical' disease any more than they can believe in fairies? A man with a leg amputated is clearly suffering from a disability – you would be hard pressed to find disagreement with that statement. But far too often and for far too long, those disabled with illness of the mind are not given the same support. What some people see is not an illness but a person who is simply angry, withdrawn, confused or hapless. The inclination is to blame the individual for having a weakness of their personality or stature. The knee jerk reaction is to want them to stop being lazy and 'pull themselves together'. Once again, the devil that is the disease escapes any form of scrutiny or challenge.

As a clinician, mental illness seems to occupy this almost impossible position of blinding the sufferer and being ignored by society though the disbelief in its very existence. How do you fight such a formidable enemy? Well, thankfully it does have its weakness. And we can exploit this weakness and fight the very thing that keeps it so elusive. We can start to banish miseducation and misconception. When we see it for what it is – an illness no different to diabetes or heart disease – we can demystify and beat it. The aim of this book was set out in the introduction, and if it achieves this aim, depression will never be as mystical again and the hope is that those suffering will see their illness conquered.

I hope that by reading this chapter, the concept of depression and anxiety has become a little clearer. There is still much to discuss about this subject. But we could not possibly begin to beat this disease before we see it and understand it. But before that we need to believe in it.

Hopefully soon we, as a society, will start to believe in, see, understand and finally beat depression.

HOW BAD CAN DEPRESSION GET?

"I don't like standing near the edge of a platform when an express train is passing through. I like to stand right back and if possible get a pillar between me and the train. I don't like to stand by the side of a ship and look down into the water. A second's action would end everything. A few drops of desperation."

- *Winston Churchill (1874-1965)*

We have spent a little time now talking about the fact that depression is a real-life illness with real symptoms and consequences. When asked to think about deadly diseases, there are certain illnesses that often spring to mind. AIDS, heart failure, meningitis, cancer – to name a few. Depression, as an illness, rarely gets a mention in a list like that.

Cause of death in the population varies with age. As we get older, the chances of dying from heart disease, cancer or stroke becomes exponentially higher. But what about causes of death in younger people?

In the UK, the Office for National Statistics publishes annual data for causes of death in different age groups. In males, in the 5-19 age group, suicide is the second biggest killer (after road traffic accidents), in the 20-34 age group, suicide is the biggest killer and in the 35-49 age group, suicide is the biggest killer. In the 50-64 age group, suicide is the seventh biggest killer.

Why is it that when presented with these unequivocally sombre statistics we still do not see depression for what it is? It is in fact the biggest killer of young adults in the Western world. Despite this, its profile in the public domain remains far lower than for cancer or, for example, heart disease. This needs to change. No other illness that causes this much mortality occupies such an inconspicuous position in the public profile. It's almost as though we are wilfully ignoring it as an entity. Depression, as we have discussed, is an illness. Now we will see just how serious an illness it can be.

In medicine, we talk about mortality and morbidity.

Mortality refers to the end of life and its cause. In the form of suicide, depression has a clear-cut mortality associated with it. However, morbidity refers to the whole collection of disabling effects that an illness can produce. The morbidity associated with the illness is vast and almost impossible to estimate.

THE MORBIDITY OF DEPRESSION

Depression itself has been found to be a risk factor for a number of other illnesses. Type 2 diabetes and cardiovascular disease are higher in patients who suffer from depression – this is even after things like smoking and lifestyle factors are taken into account. No-one is really entirely sure why this association exists but there are a number of theories. It could be that there is another 'confounding' factor. For example, it could be that people with depression are less likely to take certain symptoms seriously and act upon them, whereas the same person who doesn't suffer from depression may seek medical help earlier. In this example the depression is not the direct cause of the increased morbidity but a proxy for another effect. However, there has been some research that shows that even after taking these factors into account, there are certain illnesses that are more prevalent in those that suffer with mental health issues. Is the same underlying pathology that causes depression also partly responsible for the development of diabetes? We don't know the answer to this yet, but the association is very clear.

There is a huge economic cost to depression. Some surveys have estimated that the total financial burden is up to $45 billion in the US alone. In addition to considerable pain and suffering that interfere with individual functioning, depression affects those who care about the ill person, sometimes destroying family relationships or work dynamics between the patient and others. Therefore, the human cost in suffering cannot be overestimated.

Other illness can be strongly associated with depression and anxiety. It is increasingly known that patients with diseases of the lung, such as asthma or emphysema, who also suffer with anxiety report much higher levels of symptoms than patients with the same illness who do not have anxiety. Pain sensation is very strongly associated with depression and anxiety. In fact, treatment of mental health is a key part of any long-term pain management strategy. This is not to say that people with anxiety or depression exaggerate their symptoms. The symptoms are truly more severe. In an experiment where people are subject to an identical external painful stimulus, their level of experienced pain can be influenced by the presence of anxiety or depression. This is after all other factors such as age, sex and build have been accounted for. The illness acts as a magnifier. On a hot day, if you were to hold a magnifying glass to your arm, the sun would burn hotter on your skin. You would feel the heat more strongly, not because you were consciously acting as though the burn was stronger, but because every neural pathway that led to the sensation of pain was being stimulated harder. The extra pain is very genuine and indistinguishable from the pain of a much stronger stimulus.

The increased breathlessness of a sufferer of emphysema with depression is indistinguishable from the extra breathlessness of a person with a worse state of lung function. Mental ill health is a big factor in the overall physical health of a person. Not just in a metaphorical sense, but in a very literal one. Illness of the mind can magnify illness of the body. In fact, mental illness should really just be considered to be an extension of physical illness. For this reason, it is increasingly common that recognition of depression and anxiety is appearing on international guidelines for the treatment of disease of the lungs. Cognitive behavioural therapy, which we will discuss further in this book now plays a key role in pulmonary rehabilitation of patients with chronic lung disease. The treatment of chronic pain, e.g. the long-term back pain associated with spinal disease, is hopelessly incomplete without the adequate treatment of depression or anxiety in the sufferer. I have met countless patients that have been treated with drugs as strong as morphine that have been able to significantly reduce their pain killers dose, or even come off morphine altogether, simply by removing the magnifier. The depression treatment is the pain killing treatment.

So why is it that this mysterious association exists between symptoms of these clearly physical illnesses such as a slipped spinal disc or chronic lung disease and depression? Well, the answer is really rather straightforward.

THE PATHWAYS OF SENSATION

In explaining the phenomena, it's useful to think of an electrical circuit. Let's consider the circuit that exists to turns on the light bulb in a table lamp. We know it works because the light comes on when we flip the switch. But what about when something goes wrong? Let's think about the diagram below.

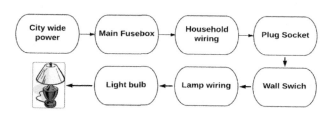

We only really have one symptom that can occur… that the light fails to come on. If the light does not come on, we know that there is something wrong. However, what we don't know is where the fault is. Because almost any fault along the necessary path to lighting the bulb will produce the exact same symptom, i.e. no light. The fault could be that the bulb itself is damaged. It may be the wiring to the bulb; it could be a fault in the switch; or it could be an electric fault in the house. In fact, even a power cut to the whole city would result in exactly the same symptom. Without further investigation, we cannot know what the cause of the bulb failure is. In this scenario, we have a relatively complex system at play to keep the bulb on, but a very simple and limited set of symptoms that the system can produce when something along the way goes wrong.

In the same way, the human brain has a limited number of external symptoms that it can display to indicate that there is something wrong. What it can't do very well is say where the problem is. Consider a very young baby; in the first few weeks of life, she has only one method of communicating… to cry. Her parents will see the same external symptom, crying, whatever the underlying cause. If she is hungry, tired, cold, hot, needing cuddles, or physically ill, the baby will have no way of communicating a state of distress other than to cry. Through care, love and getting to know the child, the parents will eventually get better and better at working out what their baby's needs are... and as any parent will tell you, this process can take a long time and there are many occasions where you just don't know.

Of course, as the baby grows, so too will her senses, and ability to communicate. She will find it easier to convey meaningful messages and her needs, her wants and her distresses will be clearer to read and see.

However, this ability to be specific about where and what the problem is does not cover all scenarios. Take pain for example. Pain is the body's alarm system. Like a car alarm, it is either on or off, but unlike a car alarm, it has levels of severity which help the individual decide how much attention to give it. Unfortunately, like our light bulb, the final pathway in the pain sensation system is limited in the number of different symptoms it can produce. Just like the light which is either turning on or not, the pain is either present or not. Just like the light bulb, whose fault could be anywhere along the circuit, the pain pathway can be stimulated at any point in its pathway and the brain will sense the exact same phenomena - pain. It is when we start to examine this pain pathway that we start to recognise why these strange associations with depression and anxiety exist.

The brain will interpret pain as originating in an area of the body. Pain will be felt in the hand, abdomen or eye, for example. All this is telling us is that the area of the brain – the sensory cortex – is displaying its alarm. Something along the path to this area of the brain has triggered a response and the brain is now consciously feeling pain.

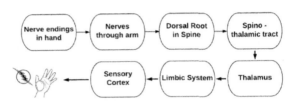

Let's consider how this pathway forms. If we think about the pain pathway from the hand, as in the diagram above, we see that it starts with nerve ending in the organ itself. Different receptors exist for different types of stimulus, namely for heat/cold sensation, for light touch and for pain. If the hand comes into contact with a noxious stimulus, such as a sharp knife, the nerve ending in this area of the body will fire off and the brain will sense pain. This is the most common, well recognised, and fairly intuitive cause of pain. However, the same pathway can be triggered further downstream.

The nerves from the hand travel up the arm and merge in the dorsal root in the vertebral column. If the nerve along this path is disturbed, the brains signal will fire in the same way – it will feel pain in the hand. Many people have heard of a phenomenon known as phantom limb pain. When a person has had a limb amputated, they no longer have that foot, arm or leg. Nevertheless, patients in this predicament will often talk about pain in the missing area of the body. This occurs because the nerve that used to arise from that part is cut further downstream at the stump. If the nerve is frayed, irritated or stimulated in any way, the brain will receive the same signal as if there were a noxious stimulus at the end of the nerve. Since the brain's sensory cortex is alerted in the same way, it will feel pain in an indistinguishable fashion. The person feels pain in a hand they don't even have.

We can follow the pathway further. Let's consider what happens at the spine. Here the nerves join the dorsal root ganglion and synapse (merge) with the spinothalamic tract which travels up the spine towards the brain. Nerves from each part of the body reach the spinal column at different points. The sensory nerves of the arm, for example, reach the spine at the neck, and the leg nerves reach the spine in the lower (lumbar) regions of the back. Just as before, a disorder at this point will produce pain in the same way. Think of sciatica. This is a pain that is felt in the buttocks and down the legs. However, a thorough examination of the legs will reveal no abnormality. The problem arises due to compression in the lumbar spine of the nerve roots that arise in those areas. Again, the brain will interpret this as pain in the area in which the nerve begins.

Now when the nerve fibres reach the brain things start to get interesting. Up until now, the messages that have arisen from the nerve endings are simply electric signals. You can think of these as the 0's and 1's passing through a digital cable to reach the intended target system. When the signal reaches the brain, it has to convert these into a meaningful sensation, which may lead to a thought or action. It remains unknown how this happens.

However, what we do know is that the nerve fibres pass through several areas of the brain – starting with the thalamus, which acts as a sort of hub – bringing in information from all senses of the body, including vision, hearing, touch, smell and taste. The thalamus starts to process the vast information that it receives every second to make it meaningful to the higher centres of the brain. This information then passes through the limbic system before reaching the neocortex. The limbic system, rather than being an individual structure, is actually a set of areas which appear symmetrically on both sides of the brain and are believed to be responsible for memory, emotion, recognition and learning.   After passing through the limbic system, the signal reaches the neocortex and now the myriad of electrical signals form a sensation, thought, idea or feeling in some conscious way. This is where pain becomes a palpable entity. This is also where a person's individuality is expressed. We are the person we are due to our neocortex. It is the seat of personality and uniqueness.

So, there is a final common pathway for almost all sensory input: the limbic system and then the neocortex. And it is this area that is strongly affected by depression and anxiety. At other points in the nerves tract, from the limb to the neocortex, it may simply be physically pinched or distorted and these disturbances will produce the sensation of pain in the relevant area. However, at the level of the limbic system, the interference is far more complex.

As we will discuss later, depression and anxiety are strongly associated with depletion or disturbance of the neurotransmitters serotonin and dopamine. The limbic system is heavily reliant on these chemicals. Illness like this can cause a myriad of disturbances at this level in the brain. Since this process is so involved in sensory function of the body, depression can therefore cause a disturbance in almost any sensation. In our example of pain coming from the hand, we have seen that nerve signals at any point along the tract will produce the same underlying sensation of pain in the area of origin, irrespective of where the nerve is being compromised. It is for this reason that interference at the limbic system, by illnesses such as depression, can have the effect of causing pain. The effect may not be the whole cause of the painful sensation but it may be altering the signal - making the pain more intense, for example. In fact, almost any physical symptom that the brain can perceive can be affected by disorders of the mind and mood.

Many of us have known people to feel sick or even actually vomit before a big stressful occasion, a driving test for example. The feeling is real. The affected individual is not making it up – they feel sick in exactly the same way as any other person with nausea. However, a thorough examination and testing of this person's bowel will not reveal any abnormality. The symptom, nausea, is being generated at the level of the limbic system in the mind. It is just as real as a symptom caused by a problem in the stomach or small bowel, but it doesn't originate there. By interfering with the sensory input at the level of the brain, depression or anxiety can produce virtually any symptom.

In fact, the sensations produced by the illness of depression or anxiety are as vast as they are strange. Common physical symptoms of anxiety can be palpitations, chest pain, shortness of breath or numbness in the fingertips. However, there are cases of patients becoming blind in a portion of their vision or losing their voice entirely. Specialists in ENT (ear, nose and throat) medicine may find no physical abnormality at the voice box, but the symptoms of being unable to properly speak remain in a condition known as psychogenic dysphonia. It's tempting to say in these scenarios that there is 'nothing wrong' with the person. This is one of the most frustrating things for me to hear said about a patient's symptoms and it is sadly a phrase all too often used by medics as well as the public. A more accurate term would be that there is 'nothing wrong with the voice box'. If there was indeed 'nothing wrong at all', then the patient would not have a lost voice. This really is akin to saying that there is nothing wrong with the light bulb in the scenario that we started the chapter with. Just because there is no pathology found in the organ that seems to be displaying the symptoms, that does not mean there is nothing wrong further downstream.

So, we see that the brain is the final common pathway of many sensory inputs. And an illness of the mind can be responsible for a myriad of different physical symptoms. There still remains a stigma attached to this however. Many people would be much happier to believe there was a problem with the organ or limb than for there to be an illness of the mind. If the problem is 'in the mind' then surely they can just snap out of it, surely it's their own doing and surely it isn't a 'real' illness. Well, I really do hope that by now the last sentence sounds as ludicrous as it is.

There are very many examples of illnesses that produce physical symptoms that are not associated with pathology in the organ involved. It takes an expert opinion from a physician to properly diagnose a fault. However, if we only look in one possible part of the system we are likely to miss the correct diagnosis on many occasions.

Let's consider some of these diseases: -

Irritable Bowel Syndrome (IBS): This is a very common illness. Its symptoms can vary hugely from person to person and from time to time within the same person. Many people describe abdominal pain, bloating and bowel disturbances. It can also be associated with back pain, tiredness, a feeling of urgency to defecate along with a host of other symptoms. If the bowels are thoroughly investigated through any number of current investigative methods, such as scanning, cameras, tissue biopsies or blood tests, nothing abnormal will be found. Yet those who suffer are truly suffering. It has since been found that one of the best treatments for this is the use of medicines that reduce anxiety or depression. Talking therapies like CBT (Cognitive Behavioural Therapy) also help. Patients find that not only do symptoms associated with thinking and the mind improve, but so does the pain in the abdomen, the bowel habit and the uncomfortable bloating. This is a truly remarkable finding and the short circuit explanation of depression or anxiety explains the associations. Here, as in the diagram for the nerves of the hand, the problem is located in the brain, with the limbic system being the most likely culprit. Hence, the solution will lie in treatment of this.

Fibromyalgia: Patients who suffer from this condition will often have joint and muscle pains. They will feel a sensation of swollen joints although they are not physically swollen on examination. Tiredness, headaches, memory loss symptoms and anxiety are common. Just like with IBS, no currently known medical test has ever been able to find any recognisable pathology in the joints or bones of these sufferers. Nevertheless, the pain is clearly real and the symptoms can be very disabling. To truly get to the bottom of the source of these issues, it is simply not enough to examine and test the joints. The rest of the system needs reviewing – including the higher centres of the brain. Again, like with IBS, the most promising treatments are based on the improvement of anxiety and depression.

Chronic Fatigue Syndrome (CFS): A great many research leads have been followed in the investigation of this bizarre illness. Previously referred to as ME, which stands for myalgic encephalomyelitis, this condition renders the sufferer with overwhelming exhaustion, muscle aches, memory difficulties and sleeping problems. Part of the diagnostic criteria for CFS is the fact that blood tests for things like anaemia, thyroid deficiency or diabetes are all negative. Just like with fibromyalgia and IBS, the organs which show the symptoms – in this case the fatigue of muscles, are not damaged in any way currently known to medical science. Yet they fail to work properly. One of the few proven effective treatments for CFS is to treat with the same medicines that treat depression. And these strategies will not only lift any psychological symptoms caused by the short circuit but also improve a host of seemingly unrelated physical symptoms, such as pain and fatigue.

It is a truly sad reflection on the state of our beliefs around illness that if the source of the physical symptoms is traced back to a problem in the brain it is considered 'not real'. Or worse, it is considered that the sufferer is somehow making it up. Worse still is the notion that the individual is entirely at fault for their own condition and that their own weakness of character has caused the problem. It is hardly surprising then, that people would much rather hear that the cause of symptoms is in an organ such as an arm, the bowel or their heart than in their most precious organ, the mind.

Part 2 - "Why do I feel the way I feel?"

WHAT IS THINKING?

"If I have done the public any service, it is due to my patient thought."

- Isaac Newton (1643 -1727)

Depression, anxiety or any other mental health disorder is fundamentally a disturbance of thinking. This is in the same sense that diabetes is a disorder of the endocrine system and pneumonia is a disease of the respiratory system.

Before we can begin to understand a disease of a bodily system we must understand the system itself. In the vast field of human medicine there exist numerous disciplines, each concerning a different aspect of this overall understanding. Anatomists, for example, are interested in the physical form of the body, its intricate layout and connections and the relevance of these to the overall function. Physiologists wish to understand the physical functions themselves – how does the body achieve respiration and gas exchange, for example. So how will we go about defining and understanding 'thought'? This is a much more elusive and difficult task than, say, the study of the kidney. The anatomy of the organ of thought – the brain - is well described; however, we are probably still many generations away from having a comprehensive theory about how this anatomical form produces conscious thought.

A huge amount of time and effort has gone into trying to understand thought, and its physical and metaphysical origins, processes, and effects. Academic disciplines as wide ranging as psychology, neuroscience, philosophy, artificial intelligence, biology, sociology and cognitive science have been involved. Thought underlies many human actions and interactions. It allows humans to make sense of, interpret, represent or model the world they experience. It allows us to make predictions about that world and mould it. To humans, who have needs, objectives, desires and plans, thought is perhaps the single most important life sustaining process.

There have been many advances in all of the fields described above, each edging us ever closer to the ultimate goal of a fully inclusive theory and understanding of the brain, consciousness and thinking. Of course, we only have the human brain as the fundamental tool of intelligence – it will remain to be seen whether it is indeed powerful enough to understand itself.

Since we will be unable to be very precise about what we mean by 'thinking' there is an element of abstraction and simplification necessary. For our purposes, we do not need to fully grasp the complex shape of the brain nor the underlying mechanisms of how it works. We are interested in the end product – the thought, the feeling or the idea. We are looking at the computer screen to understand what it is displaying without the need for the complex engineering knowledge to understand the circuit boards or the computational programming.

Let us start with something fairly straightforward and familiar. The process of thinking will tend to involve a number of steps. Firstly, we sense what is happening around us, we then process this and then compare it in our minds to our stored information (memory) before forming an analysis. This analysis will then determine our judgement of the situation and inform our bodies of what to do about it.

1. Our eyes see that water is falling from the sky.
2. Our memory knows this – we call this 'rain'.
3. We need to leave the house to go shopping.
4. This will make us wet and cold.
5. We decide to take a coat and umbrella.

This is a very simple example. You can see that it is a stepwise process. Millions of these processes will be going on in the brain and most will be on a subconscious level. Relatively few at any one time will occupy the 'higher' centres of the brain of conscious thought - few of us can handle more than a small handful on a conscious level at a time.

However, there must be more to it than this. We all think and behave differently. If it was a dry, clinical logical process then we would expect the same outcome for all people – assuming that their past experience and memory banks were approximately the same. But this is not the case. No two people respond to any one given situation in the same way. Even if the eventual outcomes are the same, each person will have a different way of interpreting the reality of a situation and might have a different way of processing the data and coming up with their own conclusion.

In fact the same person in the exact same situation may think and behave differently at different times. We can all think of times when we know that we have encountered something before but somehow responded very differently. Let's imagine a salesman who is late for work due to a traffic jam. He or she might have been in this exact position a number of times before. Each time the stakes were the same: an angry boss, a disappointed customer or an irritated colleague. But there will be times when this scenario produces high levels of anxiety and other times it doesn't. If you were to put a number of different people in the traffic jam you would undoubtedly see a range of emotions and feelings displayed. These could range from fear or anger to nonchalance or apathy.

Our reactions are the result of our sensation of the stimulus around us, the interpretation of that stimulus, the processing of how this needs to be dealt with and, finally, an action that results from this pathway.

Let's take another example. Imagine you are at work and a co-worker walks past in the corridor and doesn't say hello. Firstly, we would have to recognise that had happened – depending on how alert and aware you were you may or may not have even noticed! Then you would interpret what has just happened. The range of interpretation could be fairly wide – did your colleague simply not see you? Did they deliberately avoid you? Were they just in a bit of a daydream or were they being rude? You would then go on to analyse this. This analysis could be the most fleeting of thoughts like 'they look busy' or 'she must be in a rush'. Or maybe you might attribute some meaning to what just happened – 'is it because they don't like me' or 'am I being ignored' or 'that person is just rude'. Finally, there might be some action taken. For some it would be to shrug it off as a non-event whilst others at another time might feel the need to speak to the person to find out the problem, if there was indeed a problem. We spend much of our day making these thought processes. The vast majority of these will be entirely subconscious but there will be many other times when we think about these stimuli more deliberately.

So why do we all think and behave differently? And why does the same person think and behave differently in the same situation at different times? Well, you might argue that no two situations are ever identical. Being late in a traffic jam the first time is hardly the same as having done it for the fourth time in a month. The debate about whether your colleague has just ignored you will definitely be influenced by your relationship with them the day before or the week before. When we think about depression or anxiety, we are really talking about these thought processes being affected in some way. They might be excessively negative or ruminating. They may overvalue certain possibilities over others – even though this may seem illogical. Since the end outcome will be determined by the nature of the thought process, the actions and behaviours of any one individual will be strongly influenced by the way they have analysed the events. For example, if you were to go and have a quiet word with your colleague for being mean, this would seem more reasonable if you have interpreted them as behaving rudely. If the analysis was incorrect – and the colleague simply didn't see you, then this outcome would be inappropriate and seem irrational. Each next step in the process is a logical progression from the previous, so if there has been an error along the way, this may produce a seemingly irrational outcome.

Before continuing it is worth stating at this point that I am not suggesting that the following descriptions of thinking processes are a literal statement of how the brain works. This may sound like an obvious statement but it is important to understand this. The exact physical nature of thought is unknown and in essence is likely to remain unknown for a long time. Nevertheless, it is still immensely useful to categorise and describe the behaviour of thoughts and thinking with a view to understanding the cognitive process, if not the biological or chemical.

Let's consider what might be causing this variation in thinking between people and within the same person at different times. I think it is useful to break down the factors that influence thought process issues. I call this the 3 P's - these are: the person, the pressure and the pathology.

- PERSON
- PRESSURE
- PATHOLOGY

The person refers to an individual's personality. There has been much written about personality types. We all have unique personalities. This is what makes us human. Some people are natural worriers, some have a tendency towards optimism, whilst others are shy. There is no right or wrong. We can sometimes influence our personality and there are many factors that play a part in fashioning that unique person. Genes play a key role too. There is a strong genetic basis for traits such as shyness. Even stronger emotions, such as tendency towards anger, have been shown to be able to pass genetically from parents to offspring. There is obviously nothing you can do about your DNA makeup. Life events and experiences will also shape personality. Experiences as early as a few weeks into life seem to play a part in moulding the person.

Sometimes these are obvious but other times the traits that certain experiences can bring out are less clear. For example, there have been studies which show that newborn infants who lack close physical bonding with a parent figure can be less trusting.

The second P is pressure. This refers to stress and

stressors. When our bodies and mind are under stress we behave and think differently. As I will talk about in the chapter on stress, these changes and responses are entirely necessary for our survival. If our bodies can't be stressed by stressors then we would struggle to overcome the mildest of adversity. Stress is the physical change that occurs in the presence of stressors that allows us to function normally in less than perfect conditions. Every living creature will be able to tolerate an element of stress. Evolution and natural selection has, over millions of years, ensured that only the species and groups within a species that can naturally tolerate stress have survived. The modern human, Homo Sapiens, is well designed to cope with stressors. There is a large degree of similarity between the stress responses of different people. On a physiological level we undergo the 'fight or flight' changes which raise blood pressure and prepare us for physical endurance even though modern day stressors are usually not physical challenges. There are also changes to the way we think and process data in stressful conditions, and again there is a lot of similarity between the responses of different people. We may become more likely to overvalue possible outcomes which are less favourable to us so that we can prepare ourselves for the worst. We may start making decisions more quickly and possibly less carefully. Our emotion will be heavily influenced by the second P – pressure. Most people would react with sadness and grief in the face of bereavement. Most people would feel anger if they were subject to bullying. Most people would feel defensive or frightened in the face of imminent danger. These are all normal reactions to life events.

The third P is pathology. This is illness and plays no useful role. The illness of depression or anxiety will start to have effects on emotion and thinking. Analysis of data from stimuli may become irrational and thoughts may become locked into ruminations with no perceivable benefit. The third P is something that nobody needs and this is what we mean by mental health illness. This is the part that usually needs medical intervention. If one was unaware of the existence of the third P, they might attribute their thinking to the other 2 P's. So they might attribute the problem to a person's personality – "Pick yourself up and snap out of it!" They may also look at the level of pressure and conclude that the person should not be thinking like this with that level of stress – "Come on, there are people out there with much worse problems than you".

The third P is the short circuit that we described in part one.

In reality all three P's are present together and any one individual may struggle to know which P is causing the biggest problem. At times, the pressure is very great and the person's outward behaviour and inner thoughts may mimic depression. At other times, it may be the pathology itself that is causing the lion's share of the problem. It is important to note also that these are not 3 different elements of the same thing. They are 3 very different things. For example, you should not think of the 3 P's as 3 liquids that combine in a glass to produce an overall total volume of liquid. You can't reduce or increase one to compensate for another.

It would be more appropriate to consider them 3 ingredients for a recipe. The eggs, milk and flour of a pancake for example. Although they produce an overall effect together, they have different origins and individual natures. If your pancake was ruined due to using too much flour, you would only improve it by reducing the amount of flour. If you simply reduce the amount of milk instead, your pancake would not improve!

Through a consultation with your doctor, you will be able to gain more insight into whether pathology exists. This is a diagnosis that cannot be made by reading a book. Nevertheless, there are ways of telling the difference. Certain symptoms are often very prominent in depression and anxiety and don't usually appear though pressure alone. In sufferers of anxiety, physical symptoms such as palpitations, difficulty breathing, tremors and pins and needles can be present. In depression, people may suffer from 'early morning waking', where they are woken in the night before the alarm clock and are unable to sleep again. They may also lose weight. Both pathological conditions will be associated with the short circuit symptoms described in part one such as the ruminating, concentration difficulty, memory issues, overwhelming emotion and a loss of interest in normally pleasurable activity. Both will often be accompanied by the terrible issue of loss of insight making life even less clear.

For this reason, I simply cannot overstate how important a consultation with a doctor is. Many people will have a natural and understandable desire to blame themselves or the people around them. This is effectively trying to address the first P - person. Equally understandable is the emphasis people place on the second P - pressure. However, it is crucial to understand that eliminating pathology in the first instance will be the key.

THE FOREST ANALOGY

Another way to look at the 3 P's is in the forest analogy. Let's imagine ourselves to be in a difficult place - a forest, with trees and foliage all around and the light fading. You have been in the forest before but you don't know it all that well. Looking around, there are a few familiar landmarks but you are lost. You need to find the way out and home before it gets dark.

Now you can imagine the feelings that being in this situation might evoke. Certainly you may feel afraid – I think most people would. You may even have an element of panic and insecurity. You may feel sad because you have ended up in this situation and you may have anger toward those people and those actions that have put you in the forest in the first place. Some people may even thrive off the thought of the adventure.

Most people would agree that your first priority is your own safety. If there are other people lost in the forest with you – perhaps dependants or loved ones - their safety will be paramount too. You must begin to orientate yourself and start to consider how you might find a way out and back home. Dependant on your own life skills, the resources at your disposal and the help that you get from others, you may find this task easier or harder. Certain people may cope better in these circumstances than others. Past experiences will play a role, so will your personality type. Dependant on the size of the forest and your resilience and resolve, you will eventually complete the task more or less quickly. The impact on your personal well being will also be greater or smaller, depending on all the factors described above.

Now let's consider the same scenario, but this time with an added problem. This time, you must also wear goggles which are foggy and unclear and you must wear heavy weights on your ankles. These goggles will impact on your ability to recognise your surroundings and assess any potential threats or opportunities around you. They may even distort your vision such that you can't be clear about something you have seen. The task at hand has been made significantly harder. The weights will slow down your progress further. It will require more energy and it will heighten any emotional state that you are in. Undoubtedly, you will make mistakes and the situation may get worse. You may respond to perceived threats that aren't really there and you may be led into believing that there are paths out of the forest when really it was an illusion.

Of course, getting lost in a real forest is relatively rare – especially if you live in a city. However, metaphorically speaking, many of us have been in such a forest many times in our lives. An example would be finding yourself in debt with the goal of eliminating it. It might be a diagnosis of cancer which you battle to overcome. There are countless other examples and the size of the proverbial forest may be big or small, obviously depending on the severity of the problem. Let's see how this scenario is related to depression or anxiety – and how this fits with the 3 P's.

Person, the first P, is clearly going to be a big part. Our different make-up and traits will influence how frightened, how worried and how angry we feel. In fact some people, if they are naturally thrill-seeking, may even cherish the idea of being lost in a forest. There will be, therefore, a range of emotions right from the beginning. The emotion associated with this experience is not mental illness. The emotional response is entirely rational and, to a greater or smaller extent, any human put in the same situation would display similar emotions. Humans are happy when happy events occur, they are sad as a response to sad events, they are afraid or angry when stressors are present to stimulate these emotions.

In this example, we can consider the forest and the circumstance as a 'stressor' – this is the second P, pressure. Stressors lead to stress. The mind and body will need to adapt in some way in order to suit the challenge at hand. This will lead to new emotions that would not be there if the stressor was removed. The stressor itself is not a mental illness, it is simply a set of events or predicaments that will institute stress on that person. The chapter on stress explores what stress is and how our bodies and minds are affected by its presence. Moreover, the stress itself is not a mental illness. The body and mind needs a degree of flexibility and operate in modes that are different in some way to their preferred state. The stress response is needed to be able to cope with and overcome stressors in life.

The third P – pathology - in this example is in fact the foggy goggles and heavy weights. These play absolutely no useful role in helping to overcome the burden. Whilst wearing these goggles, the person might display emotion that is irrational in relation to the real stressor. It could be argued, however, that emotional response is entirely rational if you consider the perceived surroundings. Rather than displaying a set of emotions and stress relevant to the real scenario, the person's emotion is dictated by the distorted visual input created by the goggles. Equally, the stress response may be exaggerated as the stressor is perceived differently.

This example shows how 'stress', 'emotion' and depression are three separate things and can be defined by the 3 P's. It is common sense to see that the foggy goggles are not helping the situation. They make that task very much harder and they induce stress and emotion which may be out of proportion to the situation a person finds themselves in. Those who suffer from the illness of 'depression' or 'anxiety' are wearing the foggy goggles in the figurative sense. The lack of insight by the wearer can be very strong. For the individual involved, there is no way of telling that they are wearing the goggles and their assessment of the situation may be inaccurate or incomplete by virtue of wearing the goggles.

I am often asked if there is any point in treating depression that has been brought about by stressful life circumstances. No treatment of depression can remove the stressor – it can't pay off debt or stop the sufferer's neighbours being anti social for example. These stressors will be present throughout life – some last a lifetime, others come and go. However, the treatment of depression is thought to help by removing the foggy glasses of the sufferer. The person will still have life's stressors but will now be able to deal with these stressors in a rational and productive way.

Therefore, in answer to the question about whether treatment of depression is helpful when the stressor itself is still present, the response is most certainly yes.

In times of stress and external pressure on an individual, the last thing they need is to have to wear the foggy goggles. Removal of the offending item results in the individual better able to cope with the life events that are going on around them.

As stress, depression and emotion are so intricately linked it is entirely understandable that there is a great deal of confusion about what these things really mean. I think it is often helpful to consider how much of each component contributes to the declined wellbeing of the sufferer. Where an individual is stressed, the solution will be very different to that of the individual with depression, so distinguishing stress and depression is very important and worthwhile.

It is also worth reiterating at this point that the 3 P's are three different things. Each has its own cause and each has its own treatment. However, as we have seen, the three individual items will present themselves in a very similar way and as such are very easy to confuse. On the outside, a colleague who is behaving in a troubled or forgetful way for example could be doing so due to their individual personality makeup, it could be to do with the sheer level of stress they are under or it could be that they are ill. Or, most likely, some combination of the three. In this respect many ordinary people in society may ascribe symptoms of pathology to that individual's personality. They may say "pull yourself together", or "you need to want to be happy and moping won't help". These 'suggestions' by people may be of benefit to the lazy person but they will have nothing but a very deleterious effect on the third P, pathology. You can't treat an illness of the mind by 'snapping out of it' any more than you can 'snap out' of having your heart attack.

However, having said the three are different, there is very often an association between the pressure and the pathology. This is discussed in more detail in the pressure and pathology chapters, however it is worth reflection on why these two things, although separate, will often be seen together.

THE WASP NEST

I think a useful way to think of the relationship between stress and depression is to consider the analogy of a wasp nest in your back garden.

Imagine there is a nest in the garden, however it is out of the way and for the most part you don't see the wasps. Now imagine the scene where you have a number of children playing in the garden. They will be running up and down and curiously exploring every part of the garden playing imaginative games. Now let's add some more children to the mix and some sugary drink. What was a pleasant peaceful scene is now a full blown children's party – as we all know – sheer mayhem. Now that wasp nest is suddenly much more likely to be disturbed. And once it is disturbed the mayhem will become chaos! You are now rushing around trying to provide nibbles and cake to the children, consoling the ones who have grazed their knees and cleaning up the mud that the others have brought right through your cream carpeted lounge. Anyone with children will know exactly what I mean… this is stress personified. Suddenly you find yourself stung, then stung again and then again.

The analogy may be becoming clear. The mayhem of the party is life's stress and the wasp nest is mental illness. The two things are different. One does not cause the other and both can be present or absent completely independently of each other. However, there will always be an association between the two. Anyone in this situation may well see that every time they have a children's party, or some other loud and raucous event in their garden, they end up getting stung. Just as the children in our analogy can upset the wasp nest, stress and pressure can trigger episodes of mental illness. Many people will find that clear association between stressful life events and the onset of depression. Hardly surprising then that so many people get the two things mixed up. However, sometimes the wasp nest can become aggressive even without being disturbed. You may find yourself stung without any garden party. Here the depression has occurred without a stressful life event. People will say "but I've got nothing to be depressed about." Nevertheless, the sting feels just as bad.

Equally there may be times when you can have as many stressful children garden parties as you like (not advisable – ask any parent) and there is no sting at all. The reason there is no sting now is that there is no wasp nest. In this case, stress has not triggered depression. This fact can make the depressed individual even more confused. "How did I manage the stress of all that happened last year and come out fine, whilst now I feel depressed even though I can't find anything to be depressed about?" There is a strong association between stress and depression but they are not the same thing.

Furthermore, it will often be the case that in order to address problems in thinking you have to understand which part is causing the problem. Dealing with stress will help the pressure but no amount of treating a stressor can completely resolve a problem with pathology. This is in almost exactly the same way that no amount of antidepressant medicine is going to remove the stressor of an unpaid debt.

THE 3 RUNNERS

Another useful way to look at these 3 different entities is to think about 3 runners. In this analogy, I will show how important it is to distinguish the 3 P's in order to be able to treat them effectively.

These 3 runners all start a ten-mile race. Half way through, all three stop and are unable to complete the race. However, the reasons were different in each case. The first runner stopped because he no longer had the will or ambition to continue. He said to himself, "This really isn't for me, I'm not strong enough for this". The cause of him being unable to finish was the person. He has no regrets, he simply doesn't want to run the race… nothing more to it than that and he goes away to live his life the way he wishes to.

The second runner stopped half way through exhaustion. She said to herself "I'm really strong, I do this all the time, what is wrong with me". Well, it turns out that the second runner had already run 2 ten-mile races earlier that day. She was unable to continue. The stress on her body was too much. The cause of her being unable to finish was pressure.

The third runner stopped half way through too. He said, "I'm a strong person, I'm fit, I'm prepared and I'm well rested. I have no reason to stop in this race". Well, it turns out that the third runner had developed asthma. His reason for stopping was pathology.

Although all three runners stopped, the reasons are very different. It is useless and unhelpful to assume that the solution to each runner's difficulty is the same. It might be tempting to tell the runner to pull himself together, to get fitter and stronger. Well in the first case this might well be the answer. But in the case of the other two, this stance is clearly inappropriate. The second runner is suffering the effects of stress – her body, like anyone's, can tolerate stress but over a certain amount will have very negative effects. The third runner needs treatment for an illness. Telling him to get fitter is simply not the answer. In exactly the same way, the treatment for the third runner's asthma will do nothing to help the exhaustion of the second runner nor will it help the motivation of the first runner.

Just like the goggles in the forest analogy, the asthma of the runner is a pathology that is nothing to do with their personality and is separate to the pressure they are under. It can affect anyone, 'strong' or 'weak' and it is never useful. Many people live their lives under the barrage of this pathology and blame themselves. Or worse, other people convince them that they are to blame. Life under the pathology becomes the new normal reality. Some people live like this for so long that they forget the real person underneath. If the purpose of this book is to achieve anything, it is to wrestle the real person back from the pressure and pathology. The real person is usually a strong, fit, active and happy individual. The first step in getting that person back is to recognise that the pathology that they suffer from is not derived from the person that they are.

The next few chapters deal specifically with the person-pressure-pathology axis. In particular, we need to know more about the nature of stress itself and why it is useful to have stress tolerance. We also need to know much more about the foggy goggles.

PERSONALITY AND WHO I AM

"When I am dull with care and melancholy, he lightens my humour with his merry jests."

— *The Comedy of Errors by William Shakespeare (1564-1616)*

Amongst the first to attempt to define personalities was Hippocrates, who in 400 BC, postulated the existence of four 'humours' – yellow bile, black bile, phlegm and blood. An individual's personality and temperament were thought to be altered by the relative balance of these humours. High levels of yellow bile for example would result in an angry, easily frustrated individual. A person with a relative increase of phlegm would be calm and sluggish. The cheerful and passionate were this way due to higher than average levels of blood. In fact this system of 4 humours had been adapted from an even earlier system of Indian medicine called Ayurveda. It is difficult to say with any degree of certainty why the ancient Greek philosophers came to this conclusion or if they sought any true evidence to support the theory. However, in ancient times the stature and importance of an individual was key in deciding who was right and who was wrong. Fahreaus, a Swedish physician in the 1920's, studied the human blood clotting process. He suggested that the four humours were based upon the observation of blood clotting in a transparent container which when left undisturbed for about an hour separates into four different layers. A dark clot forms at the bottom (the "black bile"). Above the clot is a layer of red blood cells (the "blood"). Above this is a whitish layer of white blood cells (the "phlegm"). The top layer is clear yellow serum (the "yellow bile").

Whatever the origin of the four humours, the theory was developed further by one of the most influential physicians of the ancient world, the Greek philosopher, Aelius Galen. Galen made many contributions to science, philosophy, medicine and surgery. His works were adopted by Greek, Roman, Persian and later Islamic physicians. From the 11th century, Islamic texts with Galen's work were translated to Latin and became the main diet for medicine in Western civilisation. It was not until the Renaissance that the dogma of Galen's teaching was finally defeated. For over one thousand five hundred years, the teachings remained unchallenged because Galen was considered one of the greatest physicians and to challenge this level of authority could make anyone very unpopular. On many counts Galen was finally proved very wrong. There is no evidence whatsoever of the existence of humours.

More changes to thinking in Europe during the Renaissance introduced the concept of individual personality. Prior to this age, in medieval Europe, a person would be defined almost in the entirety by their associations – their family, profession or guild, and their allegiance to king and country. A few details of a person – their class and social status for example – was thought to be enough to know the mind of the person. Individuals really were cogs in a machine. This notion of 'collectivity' was a little more relaxed with higher rank. The nobility, for example, could have traits that stood them apart from each other but even then, the spread of personality was assumed to be fairly narrow.

Moving into modernity, it seems almost absurd to think that we are all clones of each other or even that we should aim to be. A large body of research has gone into discovering what makes up our personality. It is not within the scope of this book to discuss personality types at length but since our personality makes up a large amount of how we feel and think, and because so many people confuse mental illness with personality flaws, it is worth devoting some consideration to this.

From the first conception of the idea of personality 'factors' in the last 19th century, to the end of the twentieth, many psychologists have worked on finding personality traits. Whilst we are all of course, individual, there does seem to be a number of patterns and clusters of personalities which show certain similarities. Modern psychology describes the 'big-five'. These 5 broad domains or dimensions of personality make up the so-called 'five factor model.' The five areas are:

1. Openness to experience
2. Conscientiousness
3. Extraversion
4. Agreeableness
5. Neuroticism

A person with a high degree of openness will be more inclined to want to have new experiences, to appreciate art and may be more creative. Conversely, an individual with lower levels will prefer familiarly and may be more conservative to change. High scores on conscientiousness indicate a preference for planned rather than spontaneous behaviour. Extroverts like to be visible in a group and like to assert themselves, the opposite, introverts, are more reserved in social situations and enjoy more time alone. Agreeableness is a measure of a person's concern for societal harmony and regard for other people's well-being. They may be more kind and trusting. In some situations, such as in the military this trait can lead to reduced effectiveness of leadership. Finally, neuroticism is a measure of a person's likelihood of displaying negative emotion, such as worry, sadness or anger.

This does not mean that all people can be described by the 'amount' of each trait they have. The individual personality of any one person is unique. The 5 traits are simply a method of roughly categorising. In the same way one could separate a collection of objects into 5 different sizes – very small, small, medium, large and very large. This does not mean that any one object in the collection is going to be exactly one of five possible sizes. Each category is a range and although the object sits in that range it's actual individual size can be different to another in its category. The true number of different personalities is almost infinite.

The most important message for this book is that there is no right or wrong with regard to personality traits. Whilst some traits will be more useful to some people in some situations, all of the traits and sub-traits exist and this is what makes us all individual. A huge body of research has gone into whether these traits predict success in the workplace or academic achievement. With regard to the workplace, only mild correlations exist. All personality types have a role. In schools and colleges, there is some association between conscientiousness and agreeableness and high academic performance and a negative correlation exists with neuroticism. However, again, all personality types have the potential for success or failure. It may be that our educational systems provide advantage to certain traits over others. Extraversion also seems to be associated with happiness levels although the reason for this is not entirely clear.

Psychologists believe that the personality has not fully stabilised until the age of thirty. In children, psychologists talk about temperament. This can be thought of as the precursor to personality. A child's temperament will have a key role to play in their eventual personality but ultimately this can change significantly as they grow into adulthood. A common question is 'Can I change my personality?' Unfortunately the answer seems to be somewhat complex to answer. Sometimes people say "I wish I was more out-going", or "I wish I could find art more interesting". The research is not entirely clear on this. It seems to indicate that we are more inclined to not change our base personality. We can however try to express other traits, but rather like a person who is left handed trying to write with the right hand, the natural inclination will always want to go back to the left.

Unlike mental illness, which is pathological and we should attempt to treat it, personality is neither right nor wrong. There isn't a perfect personality any more than there is a perfect human or a perfect meal. Perfection is subjective. It depends on the suitability to the situation and the situation is constantly changing. The world would be a very boring place indeed if we all had the same personality. In fact, it may be down to the very fact that humanity displays such a wide range of personalities that we as a species have achieved so much. It takes every type of person to create a functioning progressive society. There is nothing wrong with that.

In my own opinion, I do not believe there is a whole lot of merit in over analysing the personality. It is what it is and all personalities have their place in this world. It would be far better to strive for happiness within one's personality than to attempt to mould it to something else. Some studies have showed that the sheer effort involved in trying to fight against natural instinct can be a disparaging and all-consuming exercise. It is also important that we accept that other personalities exist. We should ensure that in our educational systems, for example, that introverts are not given fewer opportunities than extroverts.

The problem appears when depression masquerades as a personality trait. Our personality traits will be one factor in influencing our thoughts, emotions and behaviours. In the next chapter I will discuss the second important factor – pressure – the second P. But as the third P emerges, pathology, it blends with the other two. It is this imposter of personality that makes people think that their symptoms or ways of thinking are somehow to do with the makeup of their own person. Your personality is who you are. Even though personalities can be broadly divided into categories, the number of permutations and sub-categories are vast. This makes any individual's personality unique and this should be celebrated.

PRESSURE AND STRESS – WHAT IS IT AND WHY DO I NEED IT?

"Sometimes when people are under stress, they hate to think, and it's the time when they most need to think."

- Bill Clinton (1964-)

Before we go much further, let's take a moment to consider exactly what we mean by stress. If I were to ask ten people to define stress, I'm sure I would get ten different answers. One thing that is very certain is that we all have stress in our lives.

Let's consider a few different types of stress. I

remember very clearly when I was a school boy there were times when I hadn't done my homework. The following morning, when I had to hand in my books, was a nervous time. Were the standard excuses running a bit thin? Was it worth trying a new excuse and was I in for detention or would I get away with it? It all seems a bit silly and trivial thinking back on it now twenty years on! Of course, it didn't feel trivial at the time.

Stress can be far more serious than this though. Stress can relate to single specific events or a culmination of more minor events. The teacher might say he is stressed by the pressures of his workplace targets, the homeless man is stressed by the uncertainty of where he will sleep tonight, the expectant mother may find stress in finding a problem on her baby's scan. The list is endlessly long and endlessly varied. But let's stop to consider these for a while. There is actually a lot that all of these things have in common.

Imagine an airplane flying through still clouds on a perfectly straight course to its destination across a blue cloudless sky. Everything is perfectly poised for an easy journey and the plane's body glides along with no effort at all.

Now imagine the wind picking up and starting to push the plane off course in a sideways manner. The pilot then makes an adjustment to the rudder so the plane continues on its original path. Now, although the plane is doing nothing different to previously, it is under some stress. If the plane was to remain in its original perfectly balanced and relaxed state, it would no longer be on course. It is now having to contort the structure of its body to push against the wind. It is doing the same job but having to expend more energy and its body is having to push back against an antagonistic force. Happily, the plane's body is well adapted to deal with such stress and it continues.

Further into the flight, things start to get worse. The wind picks up and there is serious turbulence. The pilot has to make adjustments to the plane's controls again, this time more extreme. The plane now judders to its destination with every part of its body being pulled and pushed in ways which strain its structure. It's not that the plane's body has much choice; if it were to give in to the forces on it, it would fall out of the sky and crash. Or at least it would give up its journey if the pilot decided to change course. These external forces that make the journey more difficult are 'stressors' and the strain on the body of the aircraft making the journey are what we call 'stress'.

When we think of stress, what we are usually describing are stressors. These are the events in our lives which generate stress in our bodies. It's worth thinking for a while about what exactly is stress. Thinking about our aeroplane example, the storm was the stressor, but the 'stress' was the way in which the plane responded to that stressor in order to continue to function as normally as possible. You might imagine the plane's rudder, aileron and flaps contorting to push again the wind or its power being diverted to its emergency systems to keep it going. Well, this is an aeroplane stressed, but what is stress in a human? When real people like you or I are faced with stressors, how do our bodies respond to maintain function?

A great deal of research has been done on this subject and a great deal is known. Some of the body's stress responses seem very sensible and very necessary, but others don't seem to make much sense at all! Well, if we are going to understand why these stress responses are there, remember that these have been formed through millions of years of evolution. Homo Sapiens, humans like you and me, appeared on Earth about 30,000 years ago, and the hominoid species which takes us back to apes is hundreds of thousands of years old. The stress response is necessary to continue functioning in the face of challenging circumstances. The species really wouldn't have got very far if it didn't have the ability to handle stress! Throughout hundreds of thousands of years of the hominoid species, the stressors haven't really changed much. These would have been the need to find food and shelter. The need to find a mate and the need to fight off predators, illness and other hominoids intent on stealing the food and shelter they have fought so long for. I doubt that any of these cavemen had 'not done my homework' on their list of stressors, nor do I think many of them were given governmental workplace targets to reach! In fact, almost all of today's stressors have really only been around for the last few hundred years – a drop in the ocean compared to the time over which our human bodies have evolved. With this in mind, it's hardly surprising that the stress responses that our bodies have developed are really designed to keep us alive whilst being chased by a big cat or get us through a period of starvation or cold. So let's get onto talking about what this 'stress' really is.

THE STRESS RESPONSE

Let's take our average modern day human being with his average modern day stressor. Let's make this chap a telesales rep and let's make the stressor a boss who wants him to reach 100 sales a week or he will be sacked. How does our poor sales reps body, evolved over millions of years to run away from predators, react?

Well, his body is almost identical to that of his ancestors a few thousand years ago. It hasn't had time to evolve its physiological response, so it behaves in exactly the same way. The body's response is both amazing and jaw dropping in its complexity. The system has kept the species alive and thriving for millennia. But is it appropriate for our telesales rep? Maybe not.

Firstly, the brain recognises the stressor. It sees this as a threat to its well-being. This threat could be existential - it could threaten the life of the individual or it could mean a deprivation of liberty, material items or power. In any case, the hypothalamus of the brain, releases a hormone called corticotropin-releasing hormone (CRH). This is the first step in the stress cascade. This neurohormone is picked up at another part of the brain called the pituitary, a small stalk-like structure in the hindbrain. The pituitary gland then releases another substance, adrenocorticotropic hormone. Once this is in the blood stream, the alarms are activated. The body has been alerted that there is trouble up ahead and that it had better brace itself. The adrenal gland is next in line. This is another small gland that sits next to the kidneys on either side. Here, the hormone cortisol is released. Cortisol gets the bodies energy systems diverted to where they need to be – to the brain, the muscles and the heart. Glucose, the body's immediate energy source and key fuel is released from stores and made available through the bloodstream – blood sugar levels rise. Cortisol also suppresses the immune system. The last thing you need when you are about to have a fight on your hands is a swollen wound as your body sits down to try to repair itself – this business can wait till later. Whilst all this is going on, the sympathetic nervous system is activated with a surge of another hormone, adrenaline. The name sympathetic is derived from the fact that it connects different parts, not, as you might imagine, because it has anything to do with the concept of emotional sympathy. On activation, every fighting force of the body is engaged. The pupils of the eyes dilate to allow more light in. The heart beats faster and harder – raising blood pressure. Blood is diverted from organs such as the skin and bowel to the muscles and kidney. This is why people 'go white' when they are scared. All very impressive indeed. Within a matter of seconds, the body is primed to fight or fly.

Well, what does our telesales rep do? He doesn't run anywhere. He doesn't fight anyone. He sits down. And tries to talk to more customers. His mind has endured stress. All the physiological changes in his body are the stress, and his situation is the stressor. Unfortunately, apart from blood and glucose going to his brain, most of the changes are simply not helpful to him in his position. In reality, this stress will have an emotional effect as well as a physical one. It is rational and predictable and any person put in the same position will show the same internal changes. Imagine what would happen if we had a much narrower range of operating conditions that we couldn't tolerate stress. Humans would not have conquered and civilised almost every corner of the Earth, however inhospitable. Even in our everyday lives, we need the ability to bend and strain, to fit into the ever-changing holes that life forces us through.

So, pressure leads to stress and this can make us feel unwell. It can make us sad or worried. It can induce anything in a vast range of emotion. It can induce medical complaints such as raised blood pressure and possibly diabetes through all that cortisol.

Let's go back to the title of this chapter - *Is depression the same as stress?* The answer is most certainly no. We need stress. We use stress to our advantage. Stress is our body's way of dealing with all of the things that get in the way of achieving our aims. The human body is an incredible machine. It can perform in the most demanding circumstances. The human mind is the pinnacle of this amazing device. The strains that it can take would truly test any man-made object.

PATHOLOGY - WHAT IS DEPRESSION AND ANXIETY?

In the opening part to this book, we looked at depression in a new light - "The Short Circuit". In this chapter, we start to delve a little deeper. What is going on in the brain at a molecular level and what is the cause of this illness?

I think the best way to start this chapter is to talk about what it isn't.

In the next part of this book, we will discuss social views on depression. It is, of course, not enough to disagree with a point of view simply because it seems unsavoury or absurd. In fact, it could be argued that the views held by many people regarding mental health are perfectly well formed – if the assumptions on which they have formed their opinion were true. But let us discuss these one by one to see if the evidence matches the statement.

The 3 very common statements about depression are

1. Depression is a state of deep sadness
2. Depression is a weakness of the mind or personality
3. Depression is a state of stress

DEEP SADNESS

One very common misconception about depression is that it is a display of sad emotion.

The human species is the most intellectually and socially advanced on Earth. We are capable of a vast range of emotion. Emotion is felt as a result of circumstance, events and past memories. There is much debate about whether babies are born with innate emotion or whether this is learned through social constructs. Nevertheless, research has shown that people across the world and across cultures will show a remarkably similar emotional reaction when placed in similar situations. We can usually empathise with another person's emotion when it is rational and brought on through life events that simulate it.

Being human will necessarily mean feeling sadness, happiness, worry, love, anger, despair, loneliness and elation amongst a plethora of other emotions. When loved ones die, we feel grief, when we have no neighbours, we may be lonely. When we pass our exams we are happy and if money is tight and there are debts we worry. We express our emotions in ways which are learned through our culture and customs. The smile is a universally recognised sign of emotion and bonding between people and normally developing babies will do this within weeks of birth.

None of the emotions listed above are depression or anxiety. It could be argued that the absence of sadness in a sad situation or the absence of worry in times of danger is abnormal in itself. Having said this, one of the key symptoms of depression is excessive amounts of sadness and one of the key symptoms of anxiety is excessive worry. So how can we tell whether the sadness we feel is depression or the worry is anxiety?

WEAK PERSONALITY

The second very important thing that depression is not is a 'weak personality'. Research shows that depression affects men and women, young and old, all social classes and all types of personality. In fact there is evidence that the exact opposite may be true. People who generally carry the weight of the world on broad shoulders seem to be more at risk of depression. People who might be considered lazy, cynical or unreliable may give up with tasks sooner than the 'strong' individual. Those stronger individuals generally bare a much greater burden of stress and so may be more likely to have depression triggered.

I wonder how many people would say Sir Winston Churchill had a weak personality. If you hold the notion that depression is a sign of weakness then this is precisely what you are saying as Churchill was well documented to have suffered depression throughout his life.

'Weakness of the mind' is hardly a term you might associate with Sir Isaac Newton, nor Albert Einstein. Two of the greatest human minds that have ever graced the Earth and minds that humanity owes so much to have suffered depression.

Already the notion that depression is associated with weakness seems to be falling apart at the seams.

NATURAL RESPONSE TO STRESS

The third misconception about depression is that this is a natural human reaction to events in their lives. The natural response to stressful events can include a range of rational emotions including sadness and anger but depression is not a natural or inevitable reaction. If it were entirely true that depression or anxiety follow a predictable course with life events, we would see a vastly different distribution of cases of depression. One might imagine that all of the people living and growing up in the slums of India or Brazil would suffer depression whilst the rich, famous and comfortably off would be entirely free of the disease. There is no question that sorrow, grief and personal hardship are far more prevalent in the deprived groups, however, it simply isn't the case that more people are depressed.

I frequently hear people say "but I've got nothing to be depressed about". As we will go on to see in more detail later, depression is not in itself a consequence of events

– there does not have to be a rational hardship. This is not to say that life events do not play a part in the development of depression symptoms. They do. But these are triggers rather than causes – think of the wasps nest.

So depression is not simply the emotion of sadness, nor is it a weakness in the psyche of an individual. Nor is it the inevitable consequence of negative events. Perhaps I should move on to what depression actually is.

SO, WHAT IS DEPRESSION?

In the very first part of this book, we looked at depression as a process. Here, we will go into a bit more depth about the different aspects of the disease.

There are a number of different tests that people can do which give a probability of depression or a severity. There are certain key symptoms that doctors will look for which may indicate that a person is suffering from depression. Whilst these clearly have their uses, I feel they do little to explain and rationalise the condition to the patient. I will reiterate that depression is a physical illness – it causes an underlying change in the physiology of the sufferer. These changes can be measured and described – and, thankfully, by addressing these pathological changes, we can control the illness.

There has been much research to suggest that patients who understand their illness and their treatment go on to have much better outcomes than those that do not. Given that mental health illness, as discussed earlier, is associated with huge levels of misunderstanding, I think it would be a very good idea to start getting people to understand the issue.

The short circuit explanation is the key starting point. Depression is not a function of personality. Nor is it a natural response to stress. Depression is simply the short circuit that appears in the thought processing workflow. It can be there in any person, under any circumstance. Even without any significant or obvious stressors, the short circuit can exist and cause all of the symptoms described in part 1. This is so important to understand as it is key in explaining that this illness is a totally different thing to the individual person. A person can be strong, intelligent, happy, brave, hardworking and proud and still either suffer from depression or not. Equally someone could be weak, ignorant, miserable, cowardly and lazy and either suffer from depression or not. The two things are not connected.

Getting people to understand might be a whole lot easier

to say than to do! I suppose it would help if doctors and scientists understood depression. There are still many unanswered scientific questions and still many mysteries and paradoxes. Not a great start then, but let's try to break down a few things we do know.

Understanding an illness has many facets to it. What do we mean by 'understand'? Do we talk about the biochemistry and physiology of the disease? I.e. *What effect is it having on the structure and function of the brain? Or do we mean why does depression occur and what causes it? Or are we interested in understanding the outward effect on the person and why they have the symptoms they do?*

I think the answers to all of the questions above are important. But as a GP who has managed many patients with this illness I feel that the answer to the last question is more important than any other. In fact, as I have said earlier, I wrote this book because I felt I could contribute most to answering this particular question and the very first part to this book does just that.

Let's now look at the science!

THE MOLECULAR BASIS FOR DEPRESSION

In human medicine, discoveries are often made in a haphazard fashion. Sometimes we know the cause of a problem simply by examining patients with the illness. In other cases, we can infer from other illnesses that have a similar set of symptoms. We might guess that 'this' illness must be related to 'that' illness. Quite often, we start out knowing nothing about the illness at all, but just that certain medicines seem to work. By working backwards, you can then determine what the underlying problem must be. If you had a problem with your mobile phone, for example, but you found that the problem went away in some rooms of the house and not in others, you might quite reasonably infer that the problem is something in those rooms – perhaps some interference from other electrical items in that room.

In the same way, we know a lot about the underlying pathology of depression by looking at the way certain medicines seem to help or hinder. Reserpine was a blood pressure drug that is rarely, if ever, used now – in fact in the UK it has been withdrawn completely. Its mechanism of action was to reduce stores of neurotransmitter chemicals in the body's nerves. This had the effect of reducing the force of contraction of the heart, thus reducing the overall blood pressure that it produces. In addition to this effect, it also reduced stores of neurotransmitter in the brain. A large number of patients on this drug then became depressed.

Conversely, another drug, Iproniazid was initially developed as an anti-TB agent. It seemed to, as a side effect, lift the mood of patients who were also depressed and in some patients caused an abnormally elevated mood (mania). This drug was also known to increase the levels of certain neurotransmitter chemicals in the brain. Iproniazid never made it as a useful anti-TB drug but did come onto the market as one of the first ever antidepressants – only to be withdrawn later due to its other side effects. Many people will be reassured to know that drug safety testing in our age is far superior and more rigorous than that in the 1950s. Again, it was noted that a drug which increases the effective concentration of neurotransmitters in the brain had a direct effect on increasing mood.

These associations were too common to be pure coincidence. This led scientists to postulate that depression is related to the depletion of neurochemicals and since then a huge volume of research work has been dedicated to this. Although there is still no overarching fundamental theory which describes why this imbalance causes mood disorders, a large body of evidence now exists to say that the two are very much linked.

Humans are very precious. They cannot be experimented on, nor can they be harmed in any way to attempt to understand them. In the not so distant past, even dissection of cadavers was prohibited. This makes the process of understanding our bodies that much harder. If we were cars it would be perfectly reasonable to take apart every part of the car, lay it out, find the faulty piece and put it back together. The same process with a human would be rather more difficult – not to mention highly unethical!

Modern methods however have given us the tools to analyse the brain and nervous system in ways which were previously unimaginable and do not hurt the subject. CT scans, MRI scans and PET scan (Positron Emission Tomography) have played a part in understanding. We can now take small tissue samples and subject them to scientific analysis with drugs without having to give them to living patients. We can look at which parts of the brain are more or less active for different patients in different circumstances. Ultimately, however, the grand test of any new drug or technology is its ability to make real life people better – very few drugs ever make it to the stage where they can be ethically and safely trialled on people.

Our molecular theories of the pathology of depression started with the observation that medicines that increase the availability of certain chemicals in the brain seem to improve symptoms of depression. This led to the notion that it may well be a deficiency in these natural neurochemicals that underlies the problem. Further research has added weight to this notion. For example, in autopsies of suicide victims, there appears to be a relative reduction in the number of certain chemical receptors in the hippocampus – a part of the brain heavily involved with memory amongst other functions. These chemicals are known as neurotransmitters and the role of these is to help transmit messages through the nervous system and brain.

Below is a diagram of a neurone – the basic building block of the human brain.

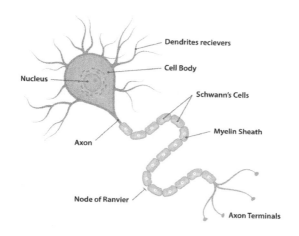

Each nerve makes connections with other nerves through its dendrites. The message is received by each individual nerve and this is transmitted through a form of electrical charge down the length of the neurone. Each individual neurone is connected to many other neurones and depending on the signal input it will then transmit the message out to other neurones which are next in line. Each individual neurone may be connected to up to 10,000 neighbouring neurones. Together this collection of neurones will make up a whole nerve or neural network. The sheer complexity of these networks is mind-boggling. Nowhere in the known universe is there such complexity – measured by number of interconnections – as there is in the human brain. It is estimated that there are 100 trillion (10 with a further 14 zeros after it!) such connections. The junction between one neurone and the next is called the synapse and that is where it gets interesting.

Whilst the message is transmitted electrically down the length of the neurone itself (the axon), when it needs to transmit to the next nerve, it does so chemically by releasing neurotransmitters.

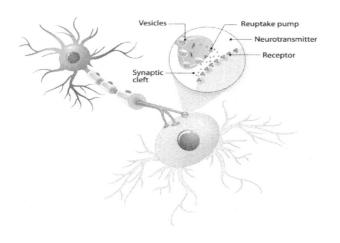

The diagram above shows where 2 neurones 'touch'. The neurotransmitters are shown as the little shapes that are released from the end of the first neurone. The second neurone has receptors which detect the presence of these chemicals and, when the transmitter is detected, the signal is passed on and continues to transmit down the next neurone which, in turn, synapses with the next.

The neurotransmitters themselves can be thought of as messengers that carry a message across the gap, delivering it at the receptor site which then acts on that message. The first neurone then reabsorbs the transmitter to use again for the next time. There are a number of different types of this neurotransmitter – the common ones being serotonin, noradrenalin and dopamine. It is these neurotransmitters that appear to be abnormal in people with mental health illness. Correction of the imbalance of these transmitters will often have the effect of improving symptoms.

Other diseases of the brain are also based on depletion of neurotransmitters. Parkinson's disease for example is characterised by the loss of dopamine in the basal ganglia system of the midbrain. Since this part of the brain is heavily involved with movement and coordination, it is these functions that the Parkinson's patient begins to lose. Parkinson's disease can also cause disorders of mood and thought – depression and anxiety being just a few examples. This in itself lends further evidence to the notion that neurotransmitters are at play in the processes of mental illness. Parkinson's disease is treated by replacement of the dopamine, amongst other modalities.

In depression, a great deal of research has been done into the role of these neurotransmitters and the current thinking is that there seems to be a relative depletion of both serotonin and noradrenaline. These two chemicals appear not to be transmitting messages across the synapse properly. It could be that there simply isn't enough of the chemical in the brain to keep up with requirements, or it could be that the receptors on the second neurone are not properly picking up the message, or it could be that the chemical is being released and then deactivated, or reabsorbed by the first neurone too quickly. One way or another, there is a physical problem with the action of the neurones which is causing some outward symptoms.

There are some holes and paradoxes in this theory though. In the section on the causes of depression, I will discuss this in more detail.

It is important to note that we don't know everything about everything. Medicine and science can be slow moving beasts, especially when applied to human beings. Nevertheless, hundreds of thousands of researchers across the globe are constantly adding little pieces of the jigsaw and every now and again the underlying picture becomes suddenly more obvious. It is a process of evolution not revolution. It is equally important not to dismiss what is known simply because we don't know it all. I have every confidence that, with time, the inner working of the human mind will become clearer. We may eventually know the exact basis by which the chemicals and cells of our brains form complex entities such as thought, consciousness and memory. But for now we don't, not fully, not even half fully. The best we can do is to look at the evidence in front of us and use this to deduce as much as we can, and by doing this a huge amount has been discovered. It requires both open-mindedness and a sense of proportion to ensure that we aren't naive about the science. Just because we don't yet have this complete fundamental understanding of the nature of thoughts, it would be absurd to not use what knowledge we do have to help those with illness of the mind in the best way we can.

It is a common misconception that illnesses such as depression are not physical – that they are brought on by an individual's personality – but research has shown beyond any reasonable doubt that this simply is not the case.

This section has introduced a chemical basis for the illness. We have already described the thought consequences of this – the short circuit. In the following sections we will consider the causes of this disruption.

THE CAUSE OF DEPRESSION

We started this book describing the 'short circuit' and in the last section, we talked about the 'chemical imbalance' as the underlying physical cause of this. Well, it's probably not quite as simple as that. In type 1 diabetes, the pancreas stops producing insulin. By replacing that insulin, you can, to a certain extent, mimic the job that the pancreas is failing to do by giving insulin injections. In hypothyroidism, the thyroid gland does not produce enough of the thyroid hormone, thyroxine. Its correction is relatively straightforward – simply replace the hormone in a pill. Once this is done to a satisfactory level, you can expect the impact on the health of the person with the under-active thyroid to be minimised. If the chemical imbalance theory of depression was as clear cut as that, you might expect to be able to conduct some form of test of the neurochemical levels to diagnose and monitor the illness. You would then expect that once the balance had been corrected, the problem would disappear. This doesn't work. Unfortunately, the true picture is a lot more complex than that.

Most psychiatrists nowadays refer to the biopsychosocial model. This doesn't give us a clear overarching cause of depression. It suggests that there are a number of factors that interact in some, as yet unknown, way to bring about the pathological state of depression. For example, our genetics play a part. Individuals in the same family as those with significant depression have a greater likelihood of suffering mental illness. This relationship persists even if related individuals grow up in very different environments. Some recent research has looked at the genes which are responsible for the receptor in the brain that deals with serotonin. There may be a link to problems in this gene and the development of illness. Like many current theories, evidence for and against has appeared and the jury is still out.

A number of other theories have been postulated. Using MRI scanning techniques, some researchers have found that the size of certain brain structures is different in those suffering depression – particularly the ventricles.

The size of the ventricles can be affected by volume of blood flow through the brain. So could there be a vascular account for the illness? Other researchers have suggested there could be an issue with the neuronal connections in the hippocampus, a part of the brain responsible for memory and mood. Neurotrophins are molecules that are responsible for the promotion of nerve development and survival. A particular form of this neurotrophin, BDNF has been found to be significantly reduced in the blood of patients who show severe depression. It is also known that anti-depression medicines have an effect on BDNF levels.

The biopsychosocial model also looks at the effect of psychology and social pressure on the development of depression and there is a great deal of literature that can be found on this topic.

It is important, I feel, to understand the subtle difference between association and cause. We currently know that there is an association between neurochemical changes and depression. We also know that there is an association between significant stressful life events and depression. But this information is not enough to say that these are the cause.

Let's take a completely made-up example of how these two things can be easily confused. Let's says that a researcher found that workers in the household cleaning products industry had a much higher rate of cancer of the lymph glands, lymphoma. If we knew nothing more about lymphoma we might assume that the products used on the factory floor were the cause. But what if it was discovered later that all those people working on the factory floor had something else in common – all the canteens for these factories were supplied by the same caterer. What if it was discovered later that it was actually the food in the canteen that was causing the problem all along. In this highly simplistic example, there is an association between working in the cleaning products industry and lymphoma. But this is simply not enough information to say that this is the cause.

Let's take a more real example. For many years, doctors would give patients with cold or 'flu like symptoms an antibiotic. The patients would get better after 3 or 4 days. Sounds like a pretty good result and it was assumed that the antibiotic had made the patient better. The antibiotic 'caused' the patient's recovery. This was until it was studied a little more thoroughly. In later decades, it was shown that patients with cold or 'flu like symptoms who didn't get any antibiotics got better in…. 3 or 4 days.

Cause and effect are very complex, especially when it comes to mental health. What is increasingly clear is that there is not one single, simple overriding cause. Or at least not one that we know about now. However, we do know of a number of significant associations. And it is because of these associations that we can start to make predictions. Just because an elegantly straightforward theory doesn't exist, that doesn't mean that we can't know plenty about an illness. It may be that searching for a cause is going to be too tough for all of us as individuals to do.

WHAT HAVE WE LEARNED SO FAR?

"The whole is more than the sum of its parts"

- Aristotle (384-322 BC)

It might be useful at this stage to start to pull things together. One of the very important messages I wish to convey in this book is the separation of the three 'P's – person, pressure and pathology. Understanding that these are 3 different entities that look very similar is fundamental to understanding what depression and anxiety are.

For example, why is it that you can be a 'strong' person

yet still suffer with depression? Why is it that you can suffer with anxiety when you have 'nothing to be anxious about'? It is perfectly understandable that people ask these questions because the 3 P's mimic each other very well. However, if we are to start the real process of getting better, we have to start to treat these three things differently. Indeed, the active and helpful treatments of these are different and it is unlikely that you will fully recover by treating one of the P's with the remedy of another.

Person - This is a personality, this is who you are. Many people will find that despite being strong individuals, they can feel depressed.

Pressure - This is the effect of stress from things that life throws at you. This is rational and will be very similar for different people put in a similar situation.

Pathology - This is illness; it can exist independent of the state of someone's personality or their stress levels.

Once this separation is made, things start to make a lot more sense. If there is pathology, this is in no way a reflection of the person. If there is significant pressure, this does not necessarily mean that there is or is not going to be pathology. Equally, if a person has a certain personality trait, this may be displayed continuously irrespective of the presence of pressure or pathology.

When I have explained these 3 separate distinct entities, my patients have often found it extremely helpful. There have been a number of occasions when patients have been brought to tears, not due to sadness, but due to the relief of finally understanding that their pathology of depression or anxiety is in no way 'their fault' or a reflection of the sort of 'person they are'. I have also found that many people are suddenly much more able to talk about mental illness more freely and openly when they understand that this is an illness, like asthma or diabetes. It is only with this understanding can we really start to beat the illness. We have exposed the devil that has been hiding himself and making people believe that it is just their own personality that is the problem.

We can now start to talk about depression as an illness like any other. It's worth having a little reflective look at some of the common things that people say about depression in this new light. I often challenge my patients to say these things out loud but instead of the word depression, replace it with the word cancer. Let's look at some of these:

"I'm not really the sort of person that gets depression" – well, as we have seen – the 'sort of person you are' is an indication of the first P, person. Whereas depression is the third P, pathology – which is an entirely separate thing.

"I'm not really the sort of person that gets cancer" – this hardly even makes sense. We are all very aware that although there maybe lifestyle risk factors to getting cancer, it is not something you get by having a certain personality.

"You need to pull yourself out of your depression" – in subsequent chapters we will learn about what treatments are available for the treatment of depression – both pill and non-pill based. However, 'pulling yourself out', is not a recognised or effective treatment.

"You need to pull yourself out of your cancer" – I'm fairly certain no one truly believes this – it is clearly nonsense.

"The only person that can cure your depression is you". Again, this misconception assumes that the person is entirely in the control of pathology – this is not the case.

"The only person that can cure your cancer is you". Clearly this statement is not true. This is also clearly an incredibly unhelpful thing to say to a sufferer of cancer.

"You think it's bad having depression? Try living with someone with it". Another common attitude that is taken by many people.

"You think it's bad having cancer? Try living with someone with it".

"I don't really believe in depression – it's all in the mind". This misconception translates to:

"I don't really believe in breast cancer – it's all in the breast". It's at best silly, and at worst highly dangerous.

The list goes on. The more we see depression and anxiety as illnesses like any other, the more ridiculous the statements sound. You really can test the validity of the pre-conception by replacing the word depression with any other illness. If it sounds silly with the word 'cancer', it's just as silly with the word 'depression'.

The second very important thing I wish to recap at this point is the notion of what depression is doing to the sufferer. This is the answer to the question – "What is the third P – pathology". We have discussed the possible neurochemical basis for depression, but what about its outward effects?

Here, it's useful to think of the 'short-circuit'. Whereas the normal process of thinking and working through problems involves a stepwise 'workflow', in depression this workflow is altered such that it goes round and round. Instead of

$$A \rightarrow B\rightarrow C \rightarrow D \rightarrow E$$

the brain goes,

$$A \rightarrow B \rightarrow C \rightarrow B \rightarrow C \rightarrow B \rightarrow C \rightarrow B \rightarrow C$$

and on and on. The process is no longer constructive. The thoughts bounce around inside the sufferer's head. The patient often knows it's happening but will find it almost impossible to turn off for any length of time. This process starts to take up so much of the person's thought process that other aspects of cognitive function suffer. Memory worsens, concentration becomes more difficult, things which are normally enjoyable cease to be so and sleep can be affected. This is amongst a myriad of other symptoms. This is the buzzing in the brain. The buzzing comes in many different forms – depression, anxiety, OCD, post-traumatic stress. The only difference is the nature of the thought that is bouncing. In depression, it is about bad things that have already happened. In anxiety, they are about bad things that might happen. The final set of symptoms the person gets is a function of the type of problem thought that is bouncing due to the short circuit.

The third and last point that I wish to recap at this stage is to do with the association of stressful life events and mental illness. If you think back to the wasps' nest analogy, this starts to make sense. Why is it that there is often a very stressful event preceding the onset of mental health problems, whereas at other times, the depression is brought on in the complete absence of stress? This is illustrated by the wasps' nest. Pressure and stress can disturb the nest that is already there (the illness) and in times of stress, the nest is much more likely to get agitated. Nevertheless, the wasps nest and the agitators are two different things. The wasps don't need the agitator to be there to become angry. Equally, if there is no nest, the person can ride through pressure and stress without any mental health illness. The two are very clearly strongly associated, however they are not the same.

Part 3 - "Why does society think the way it does?"

"THAT ROUTE"

"I told the doctor I broke my leg in two places. He told me to quit going to those places."

- Henny Youngman (1906-1998)

"I don't want to go down that route" is a phrase I hear very often indeed in my day to day job as a GP. It could be in relation to getting a diagnosis of any form of mental illness; getting treatment – pills or therapy; it being documented on the medical notes; or even that they might start considering it as a contributing factor to their symptoms.

I sometimes get a little perplexed as to what "that route" is. But a moment's consideration is probably all it needs to realise exactly what the patient is talking about. "That route" seems to be an amalgamation of all the preconceptions and judgments about mental health illness. Going down "that route" involves being labelled as 'mad or crazy', that their symptoms are 'all in the head' and that they are somehow to blame for their predicament.

Further down 'that route' would involve a stain on their records – if they were to seek help from another doctor, he or she might prejudge them as 'time wasters' or 'hypochondriacs'. Furthermore, any attempt to find new employment would be made more difficult by the fact that the new employer would see them as unreliable or 'trouble'.

Wander further down the same path and you might be faced with actually being treated for a mental illness. At this point you might be taking pills or going through counselling or therapy. The pills are seemingly particularly damning. The commonly held belief would have the patient imagine themselves to be being 'propped up' by these chemicals. Reliance and addiction would soon follow and the long struggle to 'get off' them would be far more troublesome than any short term gain they might produce. Also, the concept of any benefit is that it would be highly artificial and it certainly wouldn't address the underlying cause. They may even be dangerous in that they might mask another disease process, blinding both patient and doctor who walk together into disaster.

Counselling, depending on the patient's views, can seem even worse than the pills. This is seen as a touchy-feely technique to rid the patient of his or her 'issues'. It's useful for people who have had major trauma, physical or emotion, in their lives and if that doesn't apply to the patient then it would be a waste of time.

Well, considering all of the above, if it were true, I would certainly not want to go down "that route" either. It's difficult to imagine that any right-thinking person would willingly set off at all!

The awful shame of the situation is that none of the above are true. The truth couldn't be further from it. Yet, I can fully understand why people think the way they do about it. In reality these sorts of illnesses are common and cause huge amounts of damage to both patients and their families. And probably the worst bit of all is that it is actually very treatable in many successful ways, which are not at all harmful, and can result in people's lives being transformed.

Imagine a world in which no one would want to go down "that route" of treating asthma. Those with the condition would be so put off by the notion that they might have it and so opposed to any form of treatment that the condition simply got worse and worse. It really wouldn't be long before they started to get very ill and it wouldn't be long before people started to unnecessarily die. Even if this extreme point wasn't reached there would undoubtedly be many people whose lives were so controlled by their asthma that they could not enjoy a fulfilled life. They might be limited in their ability to exercise and engage with sport and they might start subconsciously changing their life plans to fit in with what they can and can't do. This would be a shameful situation as with the proper treatment, many asthmatics will live entirely normal lives and some asthmatics compete in the top flight of many sporting disciplines.

In the next section, I will discuss a fundamental hurdle in mental health treatment – stigma. If we are going to beat it we need to understand it. It is not enough to say that people who stigmatise are all bad – this doesn't even begin to define the complexity of the beast. Stigma needs to be eradicated. It plays no useful role in modern human society. Through analysis and recognition of the act of stigmatisation we will be best placed to defeat it.

STIGMA

"Someone has said that it requires less mental effort to condemn than to think."

- Emma Goldman (1869-1940)

The concept of stigma has some very literal roots. In ancient Greece, a stigma was a mark burned onto the body of people to signify that they were undesirable and to be avoided. This could include slaves, criminals or the insane. Like a tattoo, the mark would last a lifetime and some would try to hide it. The rest of society would often have a very negative stereotype of those branded with the stigma but amongst them would be those that were more accepting. In the modern world, we use the term stigma to mean something a little more subtle than the branding of the skin but the analogy remains remarkably appropriate and accurate. Let's consider why stigma exists.

In the study of language, it is a useful exercise to be able to compare the use and form of words across different groups and cultures. Similarities in different languages or in different groups who live separately but use the same language can be studied to trace the origin of words. A similar technique can be used to study human behaviour. When a behaviour exists in all cultures in all nations on every continent, without exception, the cause of the trait is probably evolutionary. The human smile is a universal sign, irrespective of environment, culture or ethnicity. All humans laugh, cry, form groups, suffer stress and nurture their young – amongst a vast collection of traits that cross all cultural boundaries. Even the belief in religion, a god or some supernatural phenomena has a similar cross cultural distribution that has hallmarks of an evolutionary origin. This has led to speculation that the belief in god has some evolutionary or social advantage to humans as a species. In this way, all human groups display stigmatising behaviours. All groups have stigmatised and stigmatisers. Whilst the precise form may change, the basic types of stigma remain remarkably comparable across all groups. So is this tendency to stigmatise a genetic and evolutionary phenotype that has in the past provided some advantage?

Evolution is the ultimate weed killer. Only the fittest survive. With no exception. If a trait has survived for hundreds of thousands of years, it must have been advantageous in some way or another. Unfortunately, however, that doesn't mean it is advantageous now or forever in the future. When the environment has been stable for hundreds of thousands of years and then there is a sudden change, traits that are no longer useful are most pronounced.

Take the hapless moth for example. We have all seen them fly over and over again into the light bulb – a phenomena called phototaxis. Despite getting burned they do the same thing over and over again. This trait is visible in all moths and many other flying insects. Why would they do such a dangerous and energy consuming thing. The answer to this conundrum is not fully known but may be explained through analysis of the moth's sense of direction. At night, they use the moon as a landmark or reference point. For millions of years this was the only bright light visible at night. Some moths evolved a sense of using this fixed distant object for their guidance mechanism. As the moon is very far away, the angle of flight relative to the light of the moon would stay the same throughout the flight. The method was good. It gave them an advantage over those that did not have this guidance mechanism and eventually this trait became widespread amongst the species. The planet's landscape had not changed so suddenly and dramatically for these creatures until the first human harnessed the power of fire, and then invented the candle and then the light bulb. When the moth sees a light bulb, it assumes this is the moon. Now when it flies, the angle of flight to light changes with every movement. Suddenly the directional mechanism of these insects is thoroughly confused. A genetic trait that has helped them survive as a species for millions of years is now a useless relic, completely inappropriate for the situation. Worse, it could be lethal for the moth itself. The species will evolve again and it continuously does. Perhaps not as fast as humans can change the environment though.

A number of theories have been put forward about why stigmatising may have been an advantage for early humans. In a time when sticking together in a group could mean the difference between starving to death over the winter and surviving to the spring, a sense of unity would have been vital. This unity may have been strengthened by having a sense of 'us' and 'them'. Groups that shunned outsiders or castigated certain other groups may have formed stronger bonds which helped the 'insiders' through adversity and those less inclined to form these cliques would not survive to procreate. The closed group behaviour trait would be genetically propagated and reinforced. The 'outsiders' – who were stigmatised would die – leaving more for the larger group of 'insiders'.

A similar and complementary theory is that, in prehistoric humans, quick and important judgements would have to be made about other humans in the clan based on very little information. In order to simplify it would be easier for these early humans to look for traits and make associations. As the stakes for getting things wrong would be life or death, it would be safer for them to stigmatise. If an individual has a certain trait, belongs to a certain clan or displays a certain outward appearance, they are either more or less likely to be trustworthy. In a simple cutthroat Palaeolithic past these methods of forming judgements were likely to be more effective than the more intelligent or time consuming pursuits of learning. Thus, the traits were an evolutionary advantage and passed on.

On the evolutionary scale, human society and sophistication has changed dramatically in a relatively miniscule time scale. Going from the Neolithic agricultural revolution, through the industrial revolution to the modern age of nanotechnology has taken a blink of an eye in terms of evolution. Some of the innate traits and reflexes of the cave man are as irrelevant to modern society as the phototaxic effect is to a moth flying into a lightbulb. But they are hard wired and as with many hard-wired circuits, unwiring and reprogramming is much harder work than just letting it be.

WHY IS STIGMA SO DAMAGING?

"To not have your suffering recognized is an almost unbearable form of violence."

- Andrei Lankov (1963-)

There are many illnesses which can lead to stigma. Physical deformity and disability, for example. However, mental illness seems to sit unceremoniously at the top of pile in terms of stigmatised illness. Sociologists talk about 2 forms of stigma – actual and perceived. Actual stigma is fairly obviously damaging. This is the real reaction of other people to a person with illness. The boss who victimises an employee with mental health illness or the parent who treats another person differently when their child is in their company are examples of actual stigma. Actual stigma can, and often does, result in discrimination, social exclusion and rejection. However, perceived stigma can sometimes be even more damning. A person or group of people who have experienced real stigma will go onto develop a fear and cynicism towards those that stigmatise. When the affected person walks into a room he may start to feel that unrelated and possibility innocent events are occurring because he or she is being victimised. The weight of these perceptions can be so strong that the person starts to remove themselves from society, starts to feel undervalued and may underachieve as a result.

If depression and anxiety are just the same as asthma or diabetes, then why do people think so differently about them? This is one theory.

I think a lot of it is based on how we perceive ourselves. I wonder what people would answer if they did a little thought experiment, asking themselves the question "who am I?" Try it as an exercise. Write 10 statements about "yourself", answering the question "who am I" or simply entitled "me".

It's pretty obvious that most people's answers would be fairly unique. But, I bet the answers would be related to people's personality, their thoughts and ideologies, their interests and hobbies, their jobs and their relationship with other people. If the person had some significant disability or illness, a person in a wheelchair for example, they may write about how they mentally cope with their disability. I suspect that not many people would write about the physiological state of their pancreas or the health of their lungs. People may write about their appearance and how that shapes them as a person, but I would doubt that many people would say their high blood pressure or their blood cholesterol levels defines "who they are".

Now let's have another look at the list. How many of these things are to do with the brain?

Maybe this starts to explain why we are so unaccepting of illness of the brain. If I break my arm, it's unlikely to make a big difference to "who I am". If I develop high blood pressure, again "I" haven't changed. If I get diabetes, it may make a big difference to how I might live my life but "I" am still "me".

In common perception, however, illnesses of the brain, seem to be much more personal. We can separate our physical organs from ourselves as an individual but we find it hard to do the same with our most vital organ – the brain. To have mental illness – illness affecting the higher function of the brain - seems to go to the core of a person. It's not that there is something wrong with your arm or your leg or your pancreas, there is something wrong with "you".

Is this the reason that people think differently about mental illness? If "you" are the problem then this illness is "your fault", and if you were not the way you are then you wouldn't have this illness – implying they should have control over the illness. Suddenly it becomes clearer that a misconception can domino into a huge effect and an individual can want to suppress any desire to accept the illness or get treatment in a way that they simply wouldn't do for an illness of any other part of their body.

If you stop and think about it, it seems almost ridiculous to think that disease can affect all of our other organs, but our brain – arguably the most complex entity in the known universe – should be free from any illness entirely. If the old adage is true, that the more complex a structure is, the more can go wrong, then surely we should be more accepting of illness of the brain, not less?

WHY DO PEOPLE THINK LIKE THEY DO?

I am a GP. A common or garden, jobbing general practitioner. I'm also a dad, and a husband and somebody's' son and somebody's brother. I have a daunting mortgage, a painful commute and a self-replicating daily mountain of paperwork. I also have a beautiful and kind family, a rewarding job and a lovely garden in which to relax. I get terribly upset when my lawnmower stripes on my grass aren't straight and when I'm stuck behind a learner driver. A good dinner will instantly lift my mood and my weekend can be ruined by a poor refereeing decision against my football team. I brim with pride when folk at the supermarket pour over my adorable baby girl and I get ridiculously embarrassed when in my mid thirties' I have an enormous spot on my forehead. It all sounds rather twee and obvious doesn't it – an awful set of 'first world problems'. You could get a rubber stamp and produce a whole book of 'me'.

But, of course, in reality no one knows anyone after reading a paragraph about them. We sometimes think we do. But how much of that jigsaw have we filled in ourselves? Probably a lot more than we would care to admit. There are good reasons that we do this. We are pattern recognisers. It is hard wired into our brains. Anyone that's held a baby only a few weeks old will realise that they will lock onto a human face. There is no concept of a human face in the womb so why should a face or a set of eyes, ears and a nose be anything more significant than a triangle or a blue light to a baby?

Researchers have found a part of the brain called the fusiform gyrus which seems to have areas dedicated entirely to recognising faces – it may play a part in deciphering emotion but is very likely to help us recognise people with absolute clarity even though outwardly many humans look very similar. Most of us would struggle to immediately differentiate and name five baboons in a group of forty of them, but we could pick out our family in a crowd of hundreds of thousands. Pattern recognition plays a key role in this ability. There are an almost infinite number of angles and directions that you could look at your spouse. There are an almost infinite combination of lighting and viewing conditions. There are near infinite configurations of the muscles of a person's face – the muscles they use to convey meaning through non-verbal communication, such as smiling or frowning. However, none of these really fool us; we still recognise our loved ones - instantly. And we do this through simplification and recognising a pattern. It's so instinctive that it uses virtually no effort at all.

It's only relatively recently that computers have had the power and sophistication to do the same. Border control in some countries now have computer scanners to compare a person's face to a passport photograph – but you still have to stand in a certain position, in the correct light and at the right angle before the computer can make an accurate analysis. Imagine if you had to do those computations every time you look at someone to recognise them! I get flustered with basic mental arithmetic if it involves numbers of more than one digit – but I haven't yet failed to spot my daughter when I've picked her up from nursery – no matter how much face paint or snot!

In recent years, this differential between the fast and automatic decisions and conclusions that we draw, e.g. recognising a face, and the slower thoughtful processes such as mental arithmetic, have been described as fast and slow thinking. The theory is beautifully simple. There are two channels of thinking. Each has advantages and disadvantages. Neither is always right, nor always wrong. The first channel is fast, very fast. It uses pattern recognition. The brains says "I've seen this before, I know what this is", or "I've been here before, I know exactly what to do". It is instinctive, subconscious, and automatic and we use it very often. However, it has its flaws. It might miss subtle details and differences. It might mean that a person jumps to unfair or incorrect conclusions. It may become lazy or judgmental. If the pattern recognition centres of the brain have been fed incorrect or biased information, it may result in discrimination or bigotry. But if you are driving a car and a child jumps out in front of you, you need this channel to make an instant decision – hit the brakes. Using the second channel here would result in a dead child.

The second channel is the slow channel. It takes effort, calculation and a large amount of brain resource. It is logical and unemotional and we tend to use it infrequently. The value of this channel is that it allows us to make decisions based on a more thorough analysis. It is a way of dealing with problems new to us – that we haven't encountered before. It allows us to think in new ways and can free us from pre-judgment. Its flaws, however, are obvious - it's hard work, and it's slow.

A growing body of evidence suggests that we, as humans, use the fast channel very much more often than the slow channel. This is not just limited to the everyday processes necessary to lives such as facial recognition. It also seems to encompass a wide range of decision making and opinion forming processes. Experiments have shown that even small and simple changes to the ways questions are presented can have huge impacts on people's answers. Humans seem to want to look for a pattern and make a judgement based on this. We compare what is in front of us now to something we have seen, done, heard of or learned before. And we use simple, convenient features to do the comparison. We lock on to certain aspects which we find familiar and those that fit our pre-organised fast channels.

So, when we read or hear about a person, we instinctively fill in the gaps. When we meet someone we instinctively fill in the gaps. We subconsciously know that others will be filling in the gaps about us – so we sometimes present a small part of ourselves which results in a complimentary full picture. A person who likes his lawn stripes perfectly straight must also have this personality or that way of thinking. Sulky football fans, proud dads, frustrated drivers, doctors – they all have different associations to different people – we might even call this stereotyping behaviour or pigeonholing. Or maybe it's a vital cognitive process, without which our view of what is around us would be hopelessly incomplete without every drop of detailed information. These are the pros and cons of fast thinking.

So, this brings me to question how much we really know about someone – if we have made most of it up! I suspect the system of thinking works to a greater or lesser degree because humans are a very successful species. But have we given anything up to achieve this? I think we have. Humans are nearly infinitely varied. Each one of us is different and has unique personalities. However, the number of pigeonholes in which we can sit is remarkably low.

Let's try a thought experiment. Imagine trying to recreate 'you' by going back in time. You have to create the exact person you are now with no changes. How many miniscule events have combined to produce the person you are now and the life you lead now? Everything seems so inevitable once it's done – and we only ever live out the consequences of one set of events. Perhaps there are an infinite number of universes where each of every other possibility is played out – but the one we experience is this one – and since it is the only one we know we naturally attach a level of importance to it. It is mind boggling to think how many fortuitous events would need to take place in exactly the right order to reproduce the reality of who we are, where we are and what we are.

Many people have heard of chaos theory and the popularly misquoted notion that a butterfly beating its wing can create a hurricane in another part of the world. Well of course, in a very literal sense, that is nonsense. The poor butterfly can't be blamed for the weather disaster. But what it is really saying is that in some systems tiny changes in the starting conditions, or minute differences in the conditions as the system progresses, can have a huge impact on the final result. So much so in fact that the result itself is close to impossible to predict because it is close to impossible to know the exact state of the system at the start or any other time. This might sound a little dramatic when considering human lives but the results of our infinitely varied experiences results in an infinitely varied set of people. Pigeonholing may have its uses in cognitive functioning, but it also hides and hopelessly simplifies the wonderfully complex and diverse mesh of humanity.

No matter how much simplification we apply to others though, we do know ourselves in much more detail. And, herein lies the biggest problem with this manner of viewing the world around us - that is, that we never seem to match the stereotype. And when we consider illness, this can create a deep sense of isolation – "everyone else is OK – it's just me that feels like this". The neighbours are people that 'just get on with it'; my boss is a 'doer and a maker' type; my friends are the 'sorted' type. Why am I not like that?

Well, you're not like that because they aren't either. Our minds are simply hard wired into tricking us into thinking that are like 'that'.

OPENING UP

In my role as a GP I am in a very fortunate position to be able to see much more of a person. People will open up to their doctors more so than their colleagues and sometimes their friends and family. Due to this, I will see much more than the 'stereotype'. I owe this privilege to the many generations of people before me that have worked in the NHS and given the public confidence and reassurance in those caring for them. Even if the systems and bureaucracy of this great institution are under constant fire, those staff working within it are still awarded unprecedented levels of trust from society. Doctors and nurses coming into the system recently, like me, have inherited this trust from all the hard working and dedicated clinicians that have made the NHS what it is. We have been given privileges earned by others and we must take the responsibility to uphold those values. A key value is putting the best interest of the patients and the best interests of society as a whole first.

This allows people to open up. And from the position of the listening doctor it gives a wonderfully unique insight into the difference between how people really feel and how they are perceived by others. Lots of people suffer with depression and anxiety. There isn't a 'type'. Managers, cleaners, doctors, single parents, millionaires, young, old, black, white will all present with symptoms of depression or anxiety. Many of them will feel that they are alone and their symptoms and feelings are unrepresentative of others in society in their position. This is a very great shame. Not only because it simply isn't true, but because the feeling of isolation can be the very thing that perpetuates the illness. I will often tell patients that if they were to swap positions with me for a week they would be amazed at who was consulting with the doctor for these illnesses. Even now, some people will not even talk to the doctor about their symptoms but the idea of talking freely about the illness to their colleagues or friends at the pub is unthinkable. The very individuals that people had pigeonholed into the 'sorted' category are often suffering from the very same illnesses. It's just that no one is talking about it or telling each other about it. The fundamental message of this chapter is that stereotypes don't exist. We have a fast way of thinking which is hugely advantageous in many circumstances but it has its flaws – and those are that we simplify the complex far too often. Simplification can be a good thing, but if you lose the original meaning or truth it is obviously detrimental. The upshot of this is that the preconceptions that we hold need to be challenged. Even if the sufferer of depression is not ready to openly chat about it with their peers, it is vital that the sufferer understands that they are not alone. There is a one in four chance of developing a mental illness across a whole lifetime. This means that every fourth person you walk past or speak to will have suffered the same at some point in their lives. You don't know this because they haven't talked to you about this and our brains are hardwired to categorise them into a pigeonhole which automatically makes them different to you. It is quite possible that they are thinking the same about you.

Part 4 - How do we get rid of depression?

HOW IS DEPRESSION TREATED?

One of the key messages so far has been the concept of the three P's: person, pressure and pathology. These are 3 different things which form a whole. But they are not just different versions of the same thing. You can't think of these as three volumes of water that make up the total glass. You can't compensate for an excess in one by removing some of another. They are the water, eggs and flour that make a pancake. When you look at the whole, it is very difficult to see the constituent parts. But if you are going to make corrections, you have to know which element has caused the problem.

The treatment of the 3 P's is very different. Each has a

set of modes of treatment which work. What doesn't work is treating one with the treatment of another. This is often the reason that people suffering from these illnesses fail to see any improvement in their lives. For generations, humans have treated pathology as a problem with the person. Indeed, many sufferers convinced themselves of this fact. There are personality traits which are less desirable. Laziness, apathy, selfishness and greed are just a few. If it is indeed the case that the cause of a person's outward demeanour is as a result of these traits then the 'treatment' of these is probably precisely what the typical societal view has been. *"Pull yourself together", "No-one can do this for you"* etc. There are countless books, websites and columns dedicated to helping you banish undesirable traits and develop more helpful ones. I do not wish to go there in this book. However, if the true cause of the set of external symptoms that a person feels is actually nothing to do with the 'person', then they will find that none of the 'flippant' advice given above really works. People may even find it frustrating that, despite doing everything 'right', they still find themselves under a cloud of despair or unable to enjoy the hobbies they used to enjoy.

Equally, if the problem lies entirely in the second P, pressure, an assault on the individual's personality is not going to result in any improvements. Pressure, or stress, whilst being a part of life, can be incredibly disparaging.

Again, there has been much written about the ways to reduce stress. This is important, and a good understanding of what the stressors are and the stress they cause is essential. You can't 'snap out' of having a stressor in your life. You can't mould your personality in order to reduce the debt you already owe to the bank, nor change the nuisance neighbours. Again, it is outside of the scope of this book to go into detail about how to reduce stress. However, there are numerous resources available which might be helpful depending on your own personal circumstances. As a doctor, where I feel I can help is in the eradication of pathology.

So let's talk about how we are to eliminate the third P, pathology. Since pathology is so often mistaken for personality and pressure, it is worth reiterating that no treatment for pathology will have any effect on the first 2 P's either. It is true that no amount of pills or counselling is going to make debt disappear, or make a bullying boss a nicer person. Equally, the treatments for depression will have no effect whatsoever on the personality of an individual. In reality, many people will find there are issues with pressure and pathology that need to be dealt with. It is vital to understand that both these things will need addressing if they are present. Treatment of one will not help the other and often the cause of failing to improve is that only one item was given attention and the proper treatment whilst the other was ignored entirely.

In the previous chapter, we tried to establish ways of separating out the three P's. Now we shall talk about the treatments of pathology.

Over the years, there have been many ways to treat depression and anxiety. They fall into two main categories – pills and therapies. Even within these categories there are an array of different options.

THE DRUG FEAR

"To conquer fear is the beginning of wisdom"

Bertrand Russell (1872-1970)

Medicines have always been a contentious beast. "I'm not a pill person" - is a very common phrase I hear. I've tried to break this down to fully understand what it means. On the face of it, it seems pretty self-explanatory. Someone who is not a 'pill person' is one that doesn't really like the idea of using a medicine to relieve an ailment, if they can help it. But I think there is a whole world of exploration to be done here.

I did begin to wonder who the 'pill people' that so many folk talk about were. Are there people out there who enjoy 'popping pills'? Of course, there are recreational drugs which provide the user with elevated mood and a temporary sense of euphoria, before the inevitable come down and the long term negative consequences. However, I think this is a different type of drug user. Who are these people who actually enjoy using proper medicines? Who are the pill poppers that so many people are keen to ensure they are not associated with?

I have thought long and hard about this and in conclusion, I don't actually believe that such a thing exists. I don't really believe that anyone enjoys 'popping pills'. Again, other than those that are actively abusing drugs to use them for purposes for which they are not intended, I don't think I have ever come across anyone that wishes to take medicine because it is something they enjoy doing. Where there is a big difference, however, is in people's perception about what a medicine can and can't do for them, and their willingness to use it as a means of solving a problem. The word 'drug' has a certain negative connotation to it. There are many that hold a dim view of the thought of using medicines at all. I think this is worth exploring.

WHAT IS A MEDICINE?

The European Union defines a medicine as

"(a) Any substance or combination of substances presented as having properties for treating or preventing disease in human beings; or

(b) Any substance or combination of substances which may be used in or administered to human beings either with a view to restoring, correcting or modifying physiological functions by exerting a pharmacological, immunological or metabolic action, or to making a medical diagnosis"

If you really break this down, there are an awful lot of

substances that could be defined as 'medicine'. Is coffee a medicine due to the caffeine it contains which has physiological effects? Is steak a medicine due to its high iron content which can affect the function of red blood cells? Or is it only medicine when the active ingredient has been isolated and put in a pill. Many over-the-counter cold and 'flu remedies contain caffeine, are these more medicinal than the cup of tea that also contains it? Is table salt a medicine? What about water itself? All of these substances can have significant effects on the body's physiology and metabolism and can be used to restore normal function.

I think part of the difficulty lies in the fact that the term 'drug' describes a vast array of very different things. There is a tendency to apply the same labels to all substances called a drug. This is unhelpful. A drug is as varied as a mechanical tool. A tweezer for plucking eyebrows is a tool, and so is a combine harvester. In fact, a drug is just a tool. It is a means of correcting a fault or fixing a problem. It is one of a number of different tools, each with its advantages and disadvantages. No one tool is perfect for all jobs and any engineer will tell you that going about 'fixing' a fault with the wrong tool – or indeed messing with the machine at all – can have negative consequences. Just as we only use tools when necessary, so should we only use medicines when necessary. Equally, however, if there is a necessity to fix a problem, we can't possibly proceed if we banish all 'tools' from the outset. In the previous chapter, we tried replacing the word depression with the word 'cancer'. This time we will replace the word 'pill' with 'tool'.

"I'm not really a pill-person," becomes, "I'm not really a tool-person". As I have been struggling to come to terms with what a 'pill-person' is, the notion of a 'tool-person' is equally baffling.

"I'll only use a pill as a last resort," turns into "I'll only use a tool as a last resort". Clearly this is a nonsensical statement. What tool do we mean? What is so special about this tool and why is its use going to be so bad? Is doing a job entirely by hand without the use of a tool really going to be the best way?

I must stress at this point that I am neither advocating nor dismissing the use of medicines. Moreover, I wish to get across the message that medicines are a vast array of different things that come from different sources, which do different jobs and have different pros and cons. They should be thought of as tools and there are other useful tools in the treatment of illness which are not drug based. At this stage we should concentrate on learning about these tools and then using the right tool for the right job. Just as you would not use a sledgehammer to crack a nut, so would you not use certain drugs in certain situations. However, just because the sledgehammer is particularly unsuited to the job of opening nuts, really does not mean that all tools are bad and to be avoided.

The poor old 'antidepressant' seems to sit unceremoniously at the top of the pile of drugs to be avoided at all costs. What is it about this particular tool that has caused so much aversion? Well, there is no smoke, as they say, without fire. What has caused the public view of this 'tool' to be so negative? The notion must have arisen from somewhere so let us start by exploring the history of depression treatments.

THE HISTORY OF DEPRESSION TREATMENT

Thankfully the days of treatment of mental illness with exorcism is gone. However, we only have to go back 7 or 8 generations and this was commonplace. Back in pre-renaissance era, if you were suffering from depression, or melancholia, as it was known, you would often be visited by a minister of religion rather than a medicinal doctor. Treatments ranged from the horrifically inhumane to the ridiculously ineffective. Beating, skull drilling or near-drowning would be the diet for the more unfortunate. If you were lucky enough to be treated by a more forward thinking practitioner you may be prescribed bloodletting, herbs, distraction, purgatives or even marriage!

Things have, thankfully, moved on. In the late 19th and early 20th century, influential thinkers like Sigmund Freud started to develop the notion of psychotherapy and psychoanalysis. Freud's view was that these illnesses were the result of deep seated repressed emotions and personal losses. By finding these conflicts and resolving them, he and his contemporaries thought they could cure the disease which was simply a manifestation of this. These therapies did start to show some success in moderate disease but those with severe depression still had little relief. For these people, the more extreme therapies included ECT (electro-convulsive shock therapy) and lobotomy. The lobotomy was particularly ineffective and the side effects insufferable. Patients would permanently lose their personality and the higher function or thinking, planning and decision making would be severely damaged.

Through the 1950's, doctors treating tuberculosis found that a new TB drug, Isoniazid, seemed to improve the mood of patients who were also suffering from depression. This marked the start of an era where the use of medicines hugely took off. Psychiatrists were now able to offer drugs as well as the more traditional psychotherapies to their patients. Around the same time, the monoamine oxidase inhibitors were discovered (MAO-I's). The monoamines are the neurotransmitters that have been talked about in earlier chapters. The fact that these drugs had such a positive effect on the symptoms of depression lent further evidence to the fact that neurotransmitters were at fault in the illness. Sadly, all of these drugs had very significant side effects. Isoniazid was taken off the market a few years after launch due to the potential fatal toxic effects on the liver. The MAO-I's worked well, but they meant the patient was restricted in their diet as certain food caused toxic interactions and the risk in overdose to the patient was very high.

One type of medicine that is still used today is the tricyclic antidepressant which was discovered in the 1950's and brought to market later in that decade. Imipramine was the first of these drugs to be truly tested in patients with depression and the early results were encouraging. They are called tricyclic drugs because of the 3-ringed chemical structure of its molecule. These drugs were more effective and safer than MAO-I's and soon became the mainstay of treatment. However, still, they had downsides – their side effects were sometimes intolerable and in overdose they could be very dangerous. Although tricyclics are used for depression much more rarely nowadays, they have been found to be effective at much lower doses for pain relief, insomnia and irritable bowel disease, amongst a host of other illnesses. This is common in drug development – once the tool has been created, new uses emerge that were not known or obvious to begin with.

Most of these drugs were used almost exclusively by psychiatrists. If you went to see your family doctor, you would most likely present with anxiety or a 'nervous disposition'. Into the 1960's, another type of medicine was becoming available, the benzodiazepine. The medicine you would most likely have been prescribed was Valium, or diazepam. The thing about diazepam is that it works. It works very quickly and very well indeed. Within a few hours of taking a dose, anxieties are relieved and the patient feels calmer. All sounding very positive so far. But the trouble is that really all this drug is doing is numbing the senses. It dulls emotion and anxiety. It tranquilises. And as soon as the drug has worn off, the anxiety returns. Worse than that, the drug also produces what's known as tolerance and leads to addiction. Tolerance is the name given to the phenomena that the body needs higher and higher doses to achieve the same effect. When 2mg would have produced an effect initially, the same effect would only be achieved at 5mg after a period of time. Then 10mg, then 20mg. Stopping the medicine would result in withdrawal effects. Many patients became addicted physically and psychologically. Was it really worth it? Years of weaning off a drug and the pain of withdrawal all to get a short term fix. The negative effects of Valium are most notably what many people associate with the term 'antidepressant' now and its popularity for much of the 20th century is likely to be at least in part to blame for this.

In the 1980's, a class of drugs called selective serotonin reuptake inhibitors emerged on the market (SSRI's). These were considered, at the time, a medical science breakthrough. Eli Lilly, the company that brought Prozac to the mass market started in 1971 with a compound known as LY110141. It intended this to be a treatment for high blood pressure. The substance seemed to work in animals but they had a hard time getting the same results in humans. Giving up on this, the researchers tried to see if they could get it to work as an anti-obesity drug. Again, no luck. Eventually they tried it on patients with depression. At the more extreme end of the spectrum the patients did not improve but those with moderate symptoms showed almost instant success. Realising the potential to market this new medicine, Eli Lilly wanted to push this new marvel drug hard. This was the first time that a medicine for depression was given the same marketing as Coca Cola, Nike or Sony and it was an international hit. It promised to be bliss in a blister pack and was dubbed 'the happy pill'. Promoted to the world through celebrities, expensive adverts and through campaigning on the dangers of depression directly to the public, Prozac itself has earned its parent company billions. Of course, this dubious blurring of the lines between medical altruism and cold hard product promotion has led many to be suspicious.

It's hardly surprising then, that the average man or women in the street would hold a generally negative view of drugs. Is it really worth trying to treat a condition with a chemical that might cause you serious harm, that could have you addicted or is out there being pushed by a big drug company earning billions from it? Well maybe it's time to sweep aside the judgements, the promotional material and the endless column inches of journalists with their own take on the virtues and vices of medicines to take a proper scientific look at what is and is not true.

THE TREATMENT OF PATHOLOGY

So, let us move on the crux of this chapter... how do we treat pathology, now, in the 21st century?

There are many different ways of approaching the problem. No two people are the same. No two situations are the same. Even the same person in the same situation will feel differently and have different needs at different times in their lives. I cannot stress enough at this point how important it is to seek help from your doctor if you feel you need help with the treatment of depression. In fact, there is nothing in this book that can come close to the professional and personalised advice that you can get from your own doctor. Nevertheless, I do still feel that I can try to explain the current available treatments and dispel myths.

The two modalities of treatment that I have already mentioned are therapies and pills. In fact, a great deal of research has been published on both of these. They both work. On the whole, they work as well as each other and the choice of which to pursue is very individual. My only advice is to understand each before making up your mind. Many people decide to use both and this is perfectly reasonable. It is best to discuss this with your doctor and see what different services are available locally.

I shall start with talking about medicines. As I have mentioned previously, drugs are a vast array of different entities, each with different uses, pros and cons. This section is not a detailed encyclopaedia of information about each drug but I hope it will be a useful guide to what is out there and it may be useful to have some background information before speaking to your doctor.

Essentially, the drug therapies can be broken down into those that work quickly and provide instant relief and those that take longer to work but provide a long term solution.

DIAZEPAM

I have already touched on this. Diazepam still has a role to play in this day and age. It is a sticking plaster. It will help if a person is very anxious or agitated and will work quickly. There are times when such quick acting medicines are needed. However, this drug is addictive, causes tolerance in the body and produces withdrawal effects. For the most part, its use should be limited to the short term only. Many people will feel that withholding a medicine that could have such an immediate positive effect on a person's wellbeing is cruel. However, there are many instances where people have used drugs like diazepam and then wished that they had never started. The effects of this medicine are to cause drowsiness and slowness of the mind. It can be used to induce sleep or relieve agitation in people with severe pain or even respiratory distress in people with terminal illness.

Diazepam is a drug in a family of drugs called benzodiazepines. There are a number of different drugs within this class. Each of these has its own unique special role owing to its speed of onset, duration of action and strength of effect. Temazepam, a benzodiazepine drug used to help with sleep, became a commonly abused recreational drug in the 1980s and 90's due to its ability to produce a strong euphoric 'high'. Because of its negative long term effects, these drugs have minimal role to play in the long term treatment of depression or anxiety for most people. Having said this, there are no black or whites in medicine. Individual scenarios sometimes require breaking the rules and sometimes breaking the rules is the only option.

SLEEPING PILLS

Temazepam has largely been superseded by more modern sleeping pills. The so called 'z-drugs', Zopiclone and Zolpidem, are often prescribed for the short term relief of insomnia. These drugs were originally marketed as less addictive than Temazepam, but evidence since their launch suggests that actually they do have potential for addiction. Sleep is a big problem for sufferers of depression and anxiety. Many people wish to 'reset' their sleep patterns with a short course of sleeping pills. This strategy rarely works. If the sleep disturbance is genuinely short term, then the sleep pattern will naturally come back with time. If, however, the sleep disturbance is more long term, as is being driven by an illness such as depression, a sleeping pill is highly unlikely to help.

Just like diazepam, the sleeping pill will only work on the night it is taken. What happens on the next night? Either another pill is taken or the sleep disturbance recurs. Then the next night? And the next? Soon the possibility of addiction looms. And the underlying cause of the sleep disturbance is still left untreated.

There are less harsh versions of sleeping pills. A common medicine used to aid sleep is an antihistamine called diphenhydramine. In the UK this is sold over-the-counter as a drug called Nytol. Antihistamines are commonly known to help with allergies and hay fever. The old fashioned antihistamines used to have a terrible side effect of causing drowsiness. Eventually someone had the idea of taking one of the worst offenders for drowsiness, diphenhydramine, and instead of marketing it as relief of hay fever, it was sold as a sleeping pill! Antihistamines, such as this, are not thought to cause physical addiction or withdrawal effects. However, they are notorious for build-up of tolerance. Some people say that after using them for less than a week they no longer have any appreciable effect. Luckily the tolerance wears off fairly quickly too. So after a break of a week or so, the antihistamine will induce drowsiness again.

Generally speaking, sleeping pills – otherwise known as hypnotics – are useful only if there is a short term problem. If sleep is disturbed for a small finite amount of time and it can be assumed with a fair degree of certainty that normal sleep habits will resume, then it might be worth embarking on a short course of sleeping pills to get through the usual period. If, however, the insomnia is more long standing and it is caused by depression or anxiety, a sleeping pill is unlikely to be appropriate. The notion that a persistent sleep problem can be 'reset' with a few nights of hypnotic medicine is unsupported by any hard evidence and unlikely to be a successful strategy. No sleeping pill will address the underlying problem of depression and sleeping pills cannot be called 'antidepressants'.

ANTI-DEPRESSANTS

To be truly described as an antidepressant, a medicine has to have the effect of removing depression. Unlike sedatives, which simply sedate, numb emotion and induce relaxation and sleep, these medicines should remove the pathology as their primary task. Think of these as fixing the pathological problem rather than masking it. The crux of medicinal treatment for both depression and anxiety in 2016 remains the SSRI. As described above, Prozac (or fluoxetine) was the first SSRI to be brought to market in the early 80's. Now there are half a dozen SSRIs. A newer development is the SNRI drug class. These are slightly different in that they work on a slightly different neurotransmitter – noradrenalin rather than serotonin.

Probably the most important thing to say about these medicines is that they do not display the same trait of addiction forming as diazepam or sleeping pills. They do not cause drowsiness. If you are a pilot it is perfectly safe to take these medicines and fly – in fact the Federal Aviation Administration of the United States has a list of allowable SSRIs that pilots can fly on. If you are a surgeon you can safely take these medicines and operate on patients. Most people get no side effects at all from these medicines. In many respects, the SSRIs have been a true breakthrough in the treatment of depression. The downside is that they take 2 to 3 weeks to start to work. These first few weeks are most likely to be tough in that there will be little or no benefit and, if there happens to be a side effect, it will most likely appear in these weeks. There has been some evidence to suggest that the first 2 weeks can produce a dip in mood before an improvement. It is difficult to say why this might be. It has been proposed that the delay in onset of action could in itself be the cause of the drop in mood. For some people, starting an antidepressant drug is a big step and will be associated with a degree of expectation and hope. If after doing this there is still no change, it can be demoralising. Nevertheless, after the 2-3 week build up period, the medicine starts working. Most people have little or no side effects by this stage. The medicines can generally be safely used for many years. Unlike a drug like diazepam there is generally no urgency to come off these medicines. In terms of a withdrawal effect, there is usually none. However, a serotonin discontinuation syndrome has been described. Some people have complained of some degree of negative effect on discontinuing the medicine. Nevertheless, on the scale of the symptoms produced by the withdrawal of drugs like diazepam, this is very mild indeed.

Because of all the 'bad press' associated with antidepressants, sadly there exists much misinformation about these medicines. There is often an assumption that these drugs produce addiction. Many people wish to stay away from anything described as an antidepressant. The public image can be of a drug that creates an artificial 'high', only to be followed by a natural low as the body withdraws. This is true of some drugs, but not of these. It's interesting to see what the effect of SSRI's is on people who are not depressed. If it were true that these medicines lifted mood then we would expect that non-depressed people would also feel better, happier and more elated. In reality this does not happen at all. In the absence of any true pathology, the medicines will do nothing. The drugs remove pathology – they take away depression – they do not 'add in' happiness.

What I am about to say next is a fundamentally key message. People who suffer from depression feel happier after starting the medicines. They feel more normal, brighter, more energetic and more themselves.

This is not because the pill is making them like that. All the medicine is doing is removing the pathology that changed them from being that person all along. Think back to the 3 P's, and we remember that the medicine works solely on the third P, pathology. It doesn't affect pressure – the debts are still there. And it doesn't affect the person. The happier, healthier person revealed by the treatments of depression is the real person and was the real person all along. The antidepressant can't make a person happy. It is completely wrong to call these 'happy pills'. The treatment of depression will only reveal the true person and sadly that person may have been plagued by pathology for so long they don't even know who that person is anymore.

These medicines are the true 'antidepressant' medicines. Unlike diazepam or sleeping pills, they don't just do one single job – make you drowsy or induce relaxation – they work by removing the pathology.

It's worth thinking back to the chapter on pathology. What is really going on in depression, or anxiety, or any number of mental health illnesses? Remember the short circuit. Thoughts, instead of progressing from A -> B -> C -> D, are repeating themselves. There is a short circuit – it goes A -> B -> C -> B -> C -> B -> C -> B. This repeating circuit is the buzzing in the brain. The buzzing that creates mental exhaustion, that takes up resources so the person can't think properly. They can't concentrate, they can't remember things they should have remembered and they can't enjoy anything they would normally enjoy because of this constant buzzing.

The process of fixing this problem involves simply correcting the short circuit. Instead of C going back to B, it can now progress again to D. The buzzing has gone.

People will suddenly feel that they are ruminating less. The feeling can be subtle – but it's palpable. Initially, a person will look back at the day they have just had and realise that they have not been locked down in a cycle of single persistent thoughts. After a period of time they will feel themselves again. Enjoyable pastimes are enjoyable again and the pressures that life is applying are suddenly more manageable.

Sadly, these medicines are not a cure. As with so many things in medicine, a true cure simply does not exist. The illness itself can come and go in time. Sometimes the short circuit is present, sometimes it is not. As we discussed previously, stressful life events – or pressure – can induce it. The good news though is that they can be controlled.

Well these medicines sound miraculous. Are there no downsides? Of course, as with everything, there are drawbacks. Many people worry about side effects, and I don't think this is an irrational worry. I do want to take a minute to talk about the side effect leaflet that accompanies all medicines. This has always been a slight bone of contention with me and many other doctors. The side effect profile of a drug is there for a very good reason. Unfortunately, its effect on the person reading it can sometime go a little beyond what it was intended to do. In order for a symptom to be listed on the side effect profile of a medicine, an adverse reaction must have been reported in a patient taking that medicine – no matter how rare. The information has become much better presented in recent years. Most medicines will list adverse effects by how common they are. To put things into a little perspective, even the common side effects are defined as affecting between 1 and 10% of all people. Over 90% of people will not even get the common side effects. If a side effect is described as very common, it will generally affect 10% of people or more. A 'rare' side effect will be suffered by 1 in 1,000. Therefore, 999 people out of 1,000 will not suffer this effect. This is not to say that side effects do not happen, but the likelihood of these needs to be put into some perspective. It is not helpful to read the leaflet as 'these are all the things that will happen if I take this pill'. The information was never intended to be this but often it is taken as that. When you buy a new TV, it comes with an instruction manual. At the back of this manual is a troubleshooting guide. In this section, it has details of what to do if the TV's screen does not come on or what to do if the sound stops working. This does not mean that these things will happen when you buy the TV and get it home, but that they might. Who in their right mind would buy the TV at all if all of these bad things were to occur? In the same way, the side effect leaflet is a troubleshooting guide. It's not that these things will happen, but that they might.

The common side effects reported in patients who take SSRIs are listed as feeling agitated, shaky or anxious, feeling or being sick, indigestion, loss of appetite or weight loss, dizziness, blurred vision, dry mouth, excessive sweating, sleeping problems, headaches, low sex drive, difficulty achieving orgasm during sex or masturbation, difficulty obtaining or maintaining an erection (erectile dysfunction).

Wow, that is a hell of a list and thoroughly undesirable. Well, remember only between 1–10% of people get anything on this list and it tends to be mild. After a number of weeks of taking the drug, most patients have none of these side effects. However, a significant proportion complain that the sexual side effects can persist. My general advice is that if a medicine has not suited, move on. If the problem is tolerable and only present for a short while it is perhaps worth giving it a bit longer, but if you are unlucky and a medicine is causing intolerable side effects – simply choose another.

THE NOCEBO EFFECT

Most people have heard of the placebo effect. This is the positive, desirable medicinal effect produced by an entirely inert substance such as a sugar or dummy pill. The theory is that the personal expectation of the receiver of the drug is the actual reason they derive benefit rather than any possible effect of the 'drug' they have taken.

The placebo effect can be very strong. In fact, good quality medical research has to go a long way to prove that the positive outcome of a study was really down to the drug they were testing and not the placebo effect. In some fields of study, such as the relief of pain, the placebo can account for up to 30% of any benefit. For anyone to truly say that a new medicine really works, it has to be able to beat the placebo effect in a fair and thoroughly well controlled way. If researchers fail to take these effects into account, they can spuriously claim that almost any intervention has had almost any outcome. In fact, these dubious claims can sometimes make up the entirety of health 'fads' and internet miracle cures. It can be remarkably easy to make a claim and 'back it up' with research. However, only if the study is extensive, thorough, fair and takes into account all possible forms of bias can its results be taken seriously. When therapies are truly held to account like this, many of the claims they make are found not to be true at all.

I am often asked for my opinion on alternative therapies or products that are being sold in health shops or online. With the vast volume of different things on sale, I have to profess that it is impossible to keep up with everything. There are certain features of claims made that make me suspicious though. If a product claims to have been 'scientifically proven' to be a cure for this or that illness, and these claims are valid, why would they be selling it online or in a shop. Selling a produce as a proven medicine to the healthcare market of the world, as the big drug firms will testify, is a very profitable business. Millions or even billions can be made. If their product works, then a well-designed and fair study will show this. If the item works, it will show through. If

NHS doctors start to prescribe the product in the UK, the company manufacturing it stands to make a great deal of money indeed. So why is it that the people making this wonder cure are selling it online or in a small shop? The likely answer is that the 'proof' that they claim to have for the product is not proof at all and a proper fair trial would disprove their claim. No doctor would buy the marketing spiel without proper proof. So, sadly for the claimant, they don't get their product onto the world's medical guidelines and plan B is to sell as much online as they can.

In the scientific and medical world, studies are peer reviewed and anybody is given the opportunity to criticise or question the methods and findings. It is perfectly possible to try to replicate studies to see if the same results are found or if there may be more to the story. Sadly, however, even this system isn't perfect. Some research never makes it to publication and this can bias the overall impression of a drug. Drug research is difficult, ethically complex and very expensive. Someone has to pay for it and if it's likely that the outcome of a project won't result in some funding it is less likely to proceed. The system is what it is. It has produced some ground-breaking advances and medicine today is unrecognisable to that of even a few generations ago – this is in large part due to the rigorous process of evidence based testing. Nevertheless, as with anything, it's worth having a clear idea of its benefits and limitations.

Just as there is a placebo effect, there is also a 'nocebo' effect. This is the term given to the negative side effects experienced by people who take an entirely inert substance. Just as with a placebo, where a positive expectation produces a positive effect, a negative expectation can produce a negative effect. Think back to the chapter on the brain's ability to sense. All sensory input passes through the limbic system where it is processed before becoming a real-life sensation, thought or idea. By interfering with this processing, almost any sensation can be perceived by the brain. And this perceived sensation will be very real. Often indistinguishable from the effects of true noxious stimulus. In studies on the treatment of depression and anxiety, a huge number of participants that have been given the placebo pill describe side effects. The sensation of these effects is real; the brain receives signals suggesting these symptoms but they cannot possibly have been caused by the placebo pill as there was no active drug in it. The only logical explanation is that the signal to the brain has been skewed at the limbic system, or in some higher area of the brain.

It has been shown that the placebo, or nocebo, effects are more prominent where there is a certain expectation or fear before starting. As we have discussed, patients being treated with anti-depressants can have preconceptions which are far stronger than with other forms of medicine. It is hardly surprising then that nocebo effects are commonly seen. Also, the illness of anxiety itself will be heightening fear and worry. This heightened state of wariness will further add to the nocebo effect. On top of this, add the fact that the medicine is unlikely to do anything useful for 2-3 weeks. The cocktail can be very likely to produce side effects that are not necessarily true side effects of the drug at all - but are genuinely perceived by the brain as such.

Side-effects are a complex business. As we have seen, they affect different people in different ways and even the so-called common side effects can be relatively infrequently seen. There are also nocebo effects – the notion that someone can read the side-effect leaflet and then find they have the symptoms is actually relatively common. People who find themselves in that situation are not making it up – the set of symptoms they feel are as real as anyone's, but at the same time, it may not be the drug that's caused the effect either. It is fundamentally important to seek good medical advice in these situations. Between patient and doctor, there should be some attempt to decide what the cause of the negative symptoms are.

In conclusion on this topic on adverse effects, I would encourage anyone to get to see their own doctor and get a real honest opinion on what the likely dangers are or are not. There is too much misinformation and people make poor choices when they are ill informed. As a GP, many patients ask whether they should or should not take certain medicines. Clearly, there are scenarios where professional advice would be fairly clear cut on one option over another. But really I think the more appropriate method is to help the patient choose by providing good quality understandable information.

Imagine if you went into a car showroom to buy a car. The salesman comes over and gives you some information sheets about the cars on display. You go on to make a decision based on that information. It may be that you didn't buy a certain car because you thought the brakes were faulty. You may be more inclined to choose another because it has lower mileage or better fuel efficiency. Well, what if all that information was simply wrong? It's pretty unlikely you'll go home with the right car. Choosing a personal therapy, whether drug or otherwise, is no different. Once you have the tools to analyse the information presented you will make much better choices. Your doctor will be best placed to provide that quality information.

TALKING THERAPIES

Pills are not the only way of dealing with the short circuit. The so-called talking therapies have been in and out of fashion over the decades. In fact, modern scientific studies put these sorts of interventions on a par with medicinal treatments in their effectiveness in treating this condition.

In a similar way to antidepressants, counselling also seems to hold a certain preconception and prejudice amongst many people. I suspect this has much to do with the huge overuse of the term amongst Hollywood celebrities, who we imagine need to consult with their 'therapist' over every life decision. If I mention counselling as a means of treatment I do tend to get some funny looks. Many people will very quickly respectfully decline. Of those that do end up having it, most come back to say they wish they had done it years ago.

One common reason to decline the offer of counselling is the fact that the individual has good support from family, friends and neighbours. Having a social network and means of getting physical and moral support is a huge factor in determining the likelihood of any individual coming through illness. But this is different to therapy. The therapist is a professional that has a dedicated service to offer. This service is unlikely to be the same as the help and support of a friend or loved one. The two things are very important but cannot be considered the same thing. I do think that this is another failing of the communication of the medical system; that the service of counselling has been around for so long but is still considered by many to be replaceable by close family support.

Talking therapies are not for everyone. They tend to have a bigger impact on some than others. There doesn't seem to be a particular type of person that will predictably either benefit or not. For this reason I tend to suggest to all to give it a go. It does have a somewhat greater time commitment for people to give. Swallowing a pill each morning or evening is highly unlikely to consume much of anyone's diary, but to commit to an hours session on a regular basis can be troublesome for those with a busy work schedule.

It is not within the scope of this book to delve into detail about each form of therapy, but I feel it is important to understand that they are there and they do work for many people. Those with a fear of medicines may find that these forms of intervention are far more acceptable to them. These are the main forms of therapy available:-

COGNITIVE BEHAVIOURAL THERAPY

CBT is the most commonly used modern technique for many patients with depression or anxiety. It is based on the concept that thoughts, emotions and actions are interconnected. By looking at this in the context of the short circuit, CBT tries to break the cycle of ruminating thoughts by changing actions. Unlike other forms of counselling and therapy, CBT is predominantly interested in dealing with current problems. It breaks problem thoughts down into small manageable chunks which are easier to deal with than the whole overwhelming mass. It is practical in nature. It uses tools that are within an individual's grasps to start to change things that initially seem to be entirely outside of their control.

As an example - think of someone who is locked into the short circuit of the ruminating thought of feeling isolated and unloved. This then affects their actions – they do not wish to interact to go out and meet people. The overall effect is to reinforce the short circuit. By considering actions that break this cycle, the therapist can try to halt the vicious circle and repair the short circuit.

Many people say they don't like 'talking'. This form of therapy is perfectly suitable to this sort of person because it does not involve delving into their past. The techniques are pragmatic and structured, with a strong focus on practical solutions to current problems. Having said this, the therapist will not tell you what to do. Moreover, their role is to work with you to find solutions. By the end, it is hoped that the short circuit will be corrected and problem thoughts can progress in a logical fashion again.

PSYCHODYNAMIC
PSYCHOTHERAPY

Sigmund Freud, in the 1890's, started a movement that gave psychoanalysis its first serious scientific attention. He was a neurologist with a particular interest in patients affected by neurosis and hysteria. He found that many people had symptoms in organs that could not be explained by disease in the organs themselves. For example, he had patients that could not speak even though the anatomy of their voice box was perfectly normal. If you think back to the chapter on the pathways of sensation, we have explored about how any number of symptoms can be produced by illness at a higher point in the mind and doesn't necessarily obviously relate to the end organ involved.

Freud found, that by using a range of techniques that he called psychoanalysis, he was able to cure some of his patients, not only of the psychological symptoms of anxiety but also the physical symptoms too. This had become known as the 'talking cure'. Freud had numerous ideas involving dream interpretation and sexuality. Many of these have found significant criticism in the scientific community in the years after his death. Nevertheless, some of the core principles of psychotherapy have survived and endured, and certain therapy and talking based techniques have been shown to be effective in fair and robust modern clinical trials.

The key principle of this form of therapy is that you talk about your personal feelings and relationships and thoughts about other people in your life currently and from childhood. The idea is that links can be made between past events and current thoughts and actions. This can be a fairly intensive form of therapy that requires long term commitments to be successful. In the modern age, this form of therapy has diversified to include the use of music, art, drama and play. It can be applied to children as well as adults. Many people find that just the very notion of saying things out loud and being able to express feelings helps to make them feel better in a way that they didn't initially believe possible.

A benefit of doing this work with a professional counsellor, rather than a family member or friend, is that there can be no feeling of burden on the listening party. Often, telling a loved one about problems is helpful on the one hand, but then can be associated with the guilt of making them feel strained. Obviously there will be many instances of subject matter that people feel they can't talk about with friends and family for personal reasons.

HUMANISTIC THERAPIES

Humanistic therapies are based on encouragement to explore how the individual thinks about themselves. The aim is to help patients think more positively and improve self-awareness. As with all forms of therapy, there are many individual variations. A professional in this field will be able to assess and provide the best and most appropriate form of counselling for their client. Some of the aims are to create a non-judgmental environment where one can feel comfortable talking. Gestalt therapy takes a holistic approach, focusing on experiences, thoughts, feelings and actions to help improve self-awareness. This type of therapy often involves activities such as writing or role-playing.

The key is to recognise the short circuit as a fault and talk to a doctor to ascertain the best and most appropriate form of treatment.

Part 5 - How to use this book

THE CASE OF MR JAMES

This book does not style itself as self-help. The core message is to see a doctor to discuss any symptoms that you may be feeling. However, there are some key ideas which could help to make sense of what might be going on in your mind.

Let's go back to the introduction with Mr James and apply some of the things we have discussed. The delightfully colourful man had 3 components to the way his mind was thinking. These are the three P's.

The first P, his personality, was one of a strong, proud and independent man. He has served his country, served his community, served his family and taken great care of himself.

The second P, the pressure, is the collection of stressors in his life currently. Like most people, Mr James had been through tough times in his life, and like most people, he had stresses and strains in his life right now. There were some money worries, a family bust up and an ongoing problem with his physical health.

The third P, pathology, was also present. This was causing all the symptoms of the short circuit. Ruminating thoughts which produced an almost persistent metaphorical buzzing in his brain. This buzzing resulted in concentration problems, a drop in self-worth, a persistent irritability and anger. It also stopped him enjoying the things that would normally have given him so much pleasure – his garden, his grandchildren and his football team. The knock-on effect was strained relationships with family and neighbours and a slow withdrawal from society.

The problem in making the connection was the failure to spot the third P, the pathology, as present, or even that it could exist at all. Each of the outward effects on this poor man was either blamed on the second P, pressure, or brushed off as impossible due to the first P, personality.

Examples of confusing the 'person' with 'pathology':-

"I'm not really the depressive sort"
"I don't really feel sorry for myself"
"I'm not the kind of person that would allow myself to suffer depression"
"I've always been strong, I'm the one others come to for help – it's impossible for me to be depressed"

These are common ideas expressed by many people. It was certainly the case that Mr James felt this way. Fundamentally, this is a misunderstanding of the relationship between an individual's personality and their resistance to illness. Depression can affect any 'type' of person in the same way as a cold, cancer or diabetes can. It is no reflection whatsoever on the character of a person if they do or don't suffer from any form of illness. It would certainly come across as very backward in this century, to suggest that illnesses such as cancer are the fault of the individual who suffers them.

Examples of blaming the second P pressure:-

"It's hardly surprising I feel like this – look at my money problems"
"As soon as my diabetes gets sorted, I will feel better"
"Can you blame me for feeling this way with the pressure my family is putting me under"

As we have talked about earlier, there is indeed an association between life stress and the emergence of depression as an illness, but they are not the same thing. Mr James, like so many people who suffer depression will be aware, when they reflect, that there will have been times of intense stress in life which have not been associated with depression symptoms. Equally, there will have been times in life when depression or anxiety symptoms are present without any rational stressors. The two are simply different things. Many times people will put all efforts into adjusting and fixing pressures thinking that this will relieve the depression or anxiety. This may have some effect some of the time, but when true pathology exists, it can result in a very tiring and demoralising battle to ignore this and blame it all on pressures.

The third P, the pathology, or the short circuit was also there in Mr James. This bit, completely separate to the other 2 P's, was producing so many symptoms that had been ruling this man's life for many years. With society's prejudices and stigmas preventing Mr James from truly understanding the situation, this issue continued for decades.

After Mr James had looked at the short circuit explanation, things started to make sense. He could now rationalise how his symptoms were in fact not related to him as an individual. He could see how solving the pressures in his life may or may not help the pathology. And most importantly, once he saw the short circuit, he could see that it was this that was interfering with his own personality and making his pressures that much more difficult to solve.

After correction of the short circuit, through the use of medicines and talking therapies, Mr James felt himself again. This brought out the old personality that he and everyone that had known him throughout his life were used to. The anger, irritability, sleep problems, feeling of worthlessness and persistent unsolvable worry disappeared. The treatment didn't give him anything that he didn't already have. He was not 'propped up' by happy pills. The medicine helped close the short circuit and what was left was the normally functioning and good old Mr James back again. The treatment also did nothing to solve his life pressures in a direct sense. The treatment of depression does not help pay any debts or heal past relationship scars. But what it did do was allow him to think and function like himself again. Pathology, when it exists, has the effect of multiplying the effect of pressure. A relatively small problem would get stuck in the short circuit and become a big problem. A big problem would get stuck in the short circuit and become an overwhelming problem. The key to solving the situation had to start with curing the short circuit. Addressing the problems is of course important, but in the presence of a circuit that will not allow the flow of thoughts, this can be an almost impossible task.

WHAT ABOUT ME?

We come to the end of this book and if there has been anything of interest or inspiration read, then it would be worth considering if any of this applies to you. Many people will be reading this because they have been given a diagnosis of depression or anxiety and want to know more about it, or at least get some insight into explaining the strange symptoms that are associated with it. There is very good research evidence that patients who have an understanding of their illness fare much better than those who do not. It is, of course, up to the medical profession to ensure that ill people are afforded the time and patience to provide such explanations. This is easier said than done in today's heavily strained healthcare systems – but it should always be a priority. Equally, patients who take an active interest in their own health and wellbeing fare better than those who prefer to be 'looked after'.

"You're the doctor, it's up to you…" is an often used phrase and I can understand entirely why it is said by certain patients. But in reality, it is the patient, not the doctor who should be in control. The doctors remit is to explain, guide and advise and the final decisions on a course of action should be led by patient and doctor and should be acceptable to both.

As I have said in the previous chapter, if there is any definite advice or guidance that is taken from this book, it is to see a doctor that you can talk to, trust and relate to about any symptoms you may be suffering from. Nothing that you read here will in any way, shape or form replace the expert knowledge and opinion that a doctor can give to you personally about your individual circumstance. Nevertheless, I would encourage you to think about these few things which may help in forming an understanding of what might be going on.

1. Remember the 3 P's. They are separate to each other. Don't mix them up. The presence of depression or anxiety is not a reflection of strength of character and does not imply fault. This is probably one of the most key issues in people not getting better.

2. The third P is the short circuit. This can exist with or without pressure in life. It will produce a range of symptoms that will make dealing with any stressful situation much worse. Anything can get stuck in the short circuit and, depending on the nature of the stuck problem thought, the final set of symptoms can look very different.

3. Depression and anxiety are essentially the same thing. In depression, the nature of the problem thought is about bad things that have already happened. In anxiety, the thoughts are about bad things about to happen. The simple change in the nature of the problem thought in the short circuit is all it takes to produce 2 syndromes that would otherwise look like entirely different things.

4. The short circuit may also be responsible for symptoms that seem at first to be completely unrelated. Fatigue, pain, bowel symptoms, shortness of breath and sensation changes can sometimes be traced back to depression or anxiety. The limbic system and the neocortex of the brain are the final common pathway to almost all sensory input to the brain so a problem here can produce a vast array of potential symptoms. This is something that a doctor can diagnose and differentiate from other possible diseases during a consultation and work-up.

5.   Don't assume that the pathology of the short circuit can be fixed by altering problems. If depression or anxiety is there in its true sense, then it may not go away as soon as a particular event in life has passed. The short circuit itself will not be fixed by sorting out the ruminating problem that is stuck inside it. Until the circuit is fixed, another problem thought will simply get stuck.

6.   Pathology can never be fixed by criticising the person or personality. This criticism sometimes comes from others and sometimes from the person themselves – it is never helpful.

7.   The treatment of depression is often successful and may or may not involve medicines. Think of these medicines as tools to do a job. There are tools that are sometimes appropriate and at other times not. The pros and cons of the use of these tools should be discussed in a rational way to help you get the best out of them.

8.   The treatment of depression does not add anything or take anything away from personality. The happy, bright and more productive individual who has come though treatment is not this way due to the influence of medicine. In fact, that was always the real them. The illness took this away and by treating the illness, the 'real them' has returned.

DOES ANY OF THIS APPLY TO YOU?

If it does, see your doctor. If this insidious and devilish illness has caused problems in your life, you must act to stop it. It must not be allowed to continue in its invisible state, blinding both sufferer and society at large to the fact that it even exists. We must start to think of this illness in exactly the same way as any other illness. No one in their right mind would suggest that cancer is a fault of personality or that it was brought on by the way the victim him or herself thinks. No one would suggest a cancer patient pulls their socks up and snaps out of it. Like cancer, this is a lethal disease. Right now, in the western world, it continues to claim the lives of more young adults than any other medical illness. We need now, as a society, to start showing it some respect and start showing those who suffer some compassion. It is unacceptable that people feel unable to get help. If the cause of this inability was the lack of medical treatments or the lack of healthcare resources, I could understand. This is not the case. The cause is a lack of understanding and a lack of explanation. It is simply not tolerable to prolong the agony of patients, their families and the communities in which they live because of this. We have identified the problem: misinformation. Now it is time we end it.

Printed in Great Britain
by Amazon